THIS BOOK BELONGS TO:

CONTACT INFORMATION	
NAME	
ADDRESS	
PHONE #	
EMAIL	

Copyright © Teresa Rother
All rights reserved. No part of this publication may be reproduced, distributed, or transmitted in any form or by any means, including photocopy, recording, or other electronic or mechanical methods.

DEDICATION

This Tea Tasting Journal is dedicated to tea lovers who want to document their tea tasting experience.

You are my inspiration for producing this book and I'm honored to be a part of capturing the special moments of tasting, reviewing, and recording your journey.

HOW TO USE THIS BOOK

This Tea Tasting Journal will allow you to accurately record every detail of your personal experience savoring the various tea varieties. It's a great way to document tea names, origins, brewing methods, and much more.

Here are examples of information for you to fill in and write the details about your experience in this book.

Fill in the following information:

1. Date, Tea Name, Origin - Jot down the date of tasting, name, brand, seller.
2. Tea Type - Checklist for tee type (black, green, white, herbal, oolong, pu-erh, fruit, other)
3. Brewing Method - Record details of brewing method.
4. Dry Leaves - Write down amount used.
5. Water Temperature - Record water temperature.
6. Steeping time - Record the amount of time the tea was steeped.
7. Aroma - Describe the aroma when tasting the tea.
8. Liquor Color - Describe the color of the tea.
9. Liquor Taste - Describe the taste of the tea.
10. Aroma Checklist - Use the checklist to mark taste (bitter, robust, nutty, earthy, etc.).
11. Prepared With - Use the checklist to mark other ingredients added to the tea.
12. Is This Tea Good Iced - Check yes or no.
13. Purchased From - Write down where you made the purchase.
14. Would You Buy This Tea Again?
15. Ideal For - Write down food the tea pairs well with.
16. Rating - Overall rating from 1 star to 5.

TEA TASTING NOTES

DATE	TEA (NAME/BRAND/SELLER)	
COUNTRY OF ORIGIN:		PRICE

TEA TYPE

☐ black ☐ green ☐ white ☐ herbal ☐ oolong ☐ pu-erh ☐ fruit ☐ other

BREWING METHOD	DRY LEAVES (AMOUNT)	WATER TEMP.	STEEPING TIME(S)

TEA LEAVES	LIQUOR (COLOR)
AROMA	LIQUOR (TASTE)

AROMA CHECK LIST

☐ bitter ☐ robust ☐ nutty ☐ earthy ☐ citrus ☐ flowery ☐ sweet ☐ delicate ☐ malty

☐ spicy ☐ woodsy ☐ smokey ☐ other

PREPARED WITH

☐ sugar ☐ milk ☐ cream ☐ lemon ☐ honey ☐ other

NOTES

IS THIS TEA GOOD ICED?	PURCHASED FROM	
☐ yes ☐ no		
WOULD YOU BUY AGAIN?	IDEAL FOR	RATING
☐ yes ☐ no		☆☆☆☆☆

TEA TASTING NOTES

DATE	TEA (NAME/BRAND/SELLER)		
COUNTRY OF ORIGIN:			PRICE

TEA TYPE

☐ black ☐ green ☐ white ☐ herbal ☐ oolong ☐ pu-erh ☐ fruit ☐ other

BREWING METHOD	DRY LEAVES (AMOUNT)	WATER TEMP.	STEEPING TIME(S)

TEA LEAVES	LIQUOR (COLOR)
AROMA	LIQUOR (TASTE)

AROMA CHECK LIST

☐ bitter ☐ robust ☐ nutty ☐ earthy ☐ citrus ☐ flowery ☐ sweet ☐ delicate ☐ malty

☐ spicy ☐ woodsy ☐ smokey ☐ other

PREPARED WITH

☐ sugar ☐ milk ☐ cream ☐ lemon ☐ honey ☐ other

NOTES

IS THIS TEA GOOD ICED? ☐ yes ☐ no	PURCHASED FROM		
WOULD YOU BUY AGAIN? ☐ yes ☐ no	IDEAL FOR		RATING ☆☆☆☆☆

TEA TASTING NOTES

DATE	TEA (NAME/BRAND/SELLER)	
COUNTRY OF ORIGIN:		PRICE

TEA TYPE

☐ black ☐ green ☐ white ☐ herbal ☐ oolong ☐ pu-erh ☐ fruit ☐ other

BREWING METHOD	DRY LEAVES (AMOUNT)	WATER TEMP.	STEEPING TIME(S)

TEA LEAVES	LIQUOR (COLOR)
AROMA	LIQUOR (TASTE)

AROMA CHECK LIST

☐ bitter ☐ robust ☐ nutty ☐ earthy ☐ citrus ☐ flowery ☐ sweet ☐ delicate ☐ malty
☐ spicy ☐ woodsy ☐ smokey ☐ other

PREPARED WITH

☐ sugar ☐ milk ☐ cream ☐ lemon ☐ honey ☐ other

NOTES

IS THIS TEA GOOD ICED? ☐ yes ☐ no	PURCHASED FROM	
WOULD YOU BUY AGAIN? ☐ yes ☐ no	IDEAL FOR	RATING ☆☆☆☆☆

TEA TASTING NOTES

DATE	TEA (NAME/BRAND/SELLER)		
COUNTRY OF ORIGIN:			PRICE

TEA TYPE

☐ black ☐ green ☐ white ☐ herbal ☐ oolong ☐ pu-erh ☐ fruit ☐ other

BREWING METHOD	DRY LEAVES (AMOUNT)	WATER TEMP.	STEEPING TIME(S)

TEA LEAVES	LIQUOR (COLOR)
AROMA	LIQUOR (TASTE)

AROMA CHECK LIST

☐ bitter ☐ robust ☐ nutty ☐ earthy ☐ citrus ☐ flowery ☐ sweet ☐ delicate ☐ malty
☐ spicy ☐ woodsy ☐ smokey ☐ other

PREPARED WITH

☐ sugar ☐ milk ☐ cream ☐ lemon ☐ honey ☐ other

NOTES

IS THIS TEA GOOD ICED? ☐ yes ☐ no	PURCHASED FROM	
WOULD YOU BUY AGAIN? ☐ yes ☐ no	IDEAL FOR	RATING ☆☆☆☆☆

TEA TASTING NOTES

DATE	TEA (NAME/BRAND/SELLER)	
COUNTRY OF ORIGIN:		PRICE

TEA TYPE

☐ black ☐ green ☐ white ☐ herbal ☐ oolong ☐ pu-erh ☐ fruit ☐ other

BREWING METHOD	DRY LEAVES (AMOUNT)	WATER TEMP.	STEEPING TIME(S)

TEA LEAVES	LIQUOR (COLOR)
AROMA	LIQUOR (TASTE)

AROMA CHECK LIST

☐ bitter ☐ robust ☐ nutty ☐ earthy ☐ citrus ☐ flowery ☐ sweet ☐ delicate ☐ malty
☐ spicy ☐ woodsy ☐ smokey ☐ other

PREPARED WITH

☐ sugar ☐ milk ☐ cream ☐ lemon ☐ honey ☐ other

NOTES

IS THIS TEA GOOD ICED?	PURCHASED FROM	
☐ yes ☐ no		
WOULD YOU BUY AGAIN?	IDEAL FOR	RATING
☐ yes ☐ no		☆☆☆☆☆

TEA TASTING NOTES

DATE	TEA (NAME/BRAND/SELLER)	
COUNTRY OF ORIGIN:		PRICE

TEA TYPE

☐ black   ☐ green   ☐ white   ☐ herbal   ☐ oolong   ☐ pu-erh   ☐ fruit   ☐ other

BREWING METHOD	DRY LEAVES (AMOUNT)	WATER TEMP.	STEEPING TIME(S)

TEA LEAVES	LIQUOR (COLOR)
AROMA	LIQUOR (TASTE)

AROMA CHECK LIST

☐ bitter   ☐ robust   ☐ nutty   ☐ earthy   ☐ citrus   ☐ flowery   ☐ sweet   ☐ delicate   ☐ malty
☐ spicy   ☐ woodsy   ☐ smokey   ☐ other

PREPARED WITH

☐ sugar   ☐ milk   ☐ cream   ☐ lemon   ☐ honey   ☐ other

NOTES

IS THIS TEA GOOD ICED?	PURCHASED FROM		
☐ yes ☐ no			
WOULD YOU BUY AGAIN?	IDEAL FOR	RATING	
☐ yes ☐ no		☆ ☆ ☆ ☆ ☆	

TEA TASTING NOTES

DATE	TEA (NAME/BRAND/SELLER)	
COUNTRY OF ORIGIN:		PRICE

TEA TYPE
☐ black ☐ green ☐ white ☐ herbal ☐ oolong ☐ pu-erh ☐ fruit ☐ other

BREWING METHOD	DRY LEAVES (AMOUNT)	WATER TEMP.	STEEPING TIME(S)

TEA LEAVES	LIQUOR (COLOR)

AROMA	LIQUOR (TASTE)

AROMA CHECK LIST
☐ bitter ☐ robust ☐ nutty ☐ earthy ☐ citrus ☐ flowery ☐ sweet ☐ delicate ☐ malty
☐ spicy ☐ woodsy ☐ smokey ☐ other

PREPARED WITH
☐ sugar ☐ milk ☐ cream ☐ lemon ☐ honey ☐ other

NOTES

IS THIS TEA GOOD ICED? ☐ yes ☐ no	PURCHASED FROM	
WOULD YOU BUY AGAIN? ☐ yes ☐ no	IDEAL FOR	RATING ☆ ☆ ☆ ☆ ☆

TEA TASTING NOTES

DATE	TEA (NAME/BRAND/SELLER)		
COUNTRY OF ORIGIN:			PRICE

TEA TYPE

☐ black ☐ green ☐ white ☐ herbal ☐ oolong ☐ pu-erh ☐ fruit ☐ other

BREWING METHOD	DRY LEAVES (AMOUNT)	WATER TEMP.	STEEPING TIME(S)

TEA LEAVES	LIQUOR (COLOR)

AROMA	LIQUOR (TASTE)

AROMA CHECK LIST

☐ bitter ☐ robust ☐ nutty ☐ earthy ☐ citrus ☐ flowery ☐ sweet ☐ delicate ☐ malty
☐ spicy ☐ woodsy ☐ smokey ☐ other

PREPARED WITH

☐ sugar ☐ milk ☐ cream ☐ lemon ☐ honey ☐ other

NOTES

IS THIS TEA GOOD ICED?	PURCHASED FROM		
☐ yes ☐ no			
WOULD YOU BUY AGAIN?	IDEAL FOR		RATING
☐ yes ☐ no			☆☆☆☆☆

TEA TASTING NOTES

DATE	TEA (NAME/BRAND/SELLER)	
COUNTRY OF ORIGIN:		PRICE

TEA TYPE

☐ black ☐ green ☐ white ☐ herbal ☐ oolong ☐ pu-erh ☐ fruit ☐ other

BREWING METHOD	DRY LEAVES (AMOUNT)	WATER TEMP.	STEEPING TIME(S)

TEA LEAVES	LIQUOR (COLOR)
AROMA	LIQUOR (TASTE)

AROMA CHECK LIST

☐ bitter ☐ robust ☐ nutty ☐ earthy ☐ citrus ☐ flowery ☐ sweet ☐ delicate ☐ malty
☐ spicy ☐ woodsy ☐ smokey ☐ other

PREPARED WITH

☐ sugar ☐ milk ☐ cream ☐ lemon ☐ honey ☐ other

NOTES

IS THIS TEA GOOD ICED?	PURCHASED FROM	
☐ yes ☐ no		
WOULD YOU BUY AGAIN?	IDEAL FOR	RATING
☐ yes ☐ no		☆☆☆☆☆

TEA TASTING NOTES

DATE	TEA (NAME/BRAND/SELLER)		
COUNTRY OF ORIGIN:			PRICE
TEA TYPE ☐ black ☐ green ☐ white ☐ herbal ☐ oolong ☐ pu-erh ☐ fruit ☐ other			
BREWING METHOD	DRY LEAVES (AMOUNT)	WATER TEMP.	STEEPING TIME(S)

TEA LEAVES	LIQUOR (COLOR)
AROMA	LIQUOR (TASTE)

AROMA CHECK LIST

☐ bitter ☐ robust ☐ nutty ☐ earthy ☐ citrus ☐ flowery ☐ sweet ☐ delicate ☐ malty

☐ spicy ☐ woodsy ☐ smokey ☐ other

PREPARED WITH

☐ sugar ☐ milk ☐ cream ☐ lemon ☐ honey ☐ other

NOTES

IS THIS TEA GOOD ICED? ☐ yes ☐ no	PURCHASED FROM	
WOULD YOU BUY AGAIN? ☐ yes ☐ no	IDEAL FOR	RATING ☆☆☆☆☆

TEA TASTING NOTES

DATE	TEA (NAME/BRAND/SELLER)	
COUNTRY OF ORIGIN:		PRICE

TEA TYPE

☐ black ☐ green ☐ white ☐ herbal ☐ oolong ☐ pu-erh ☐ fruit ☐ other

BREWING METHOD	DRY LEAVES (AMOUNT)	WATER TEMP.	STEEPING TIME(S)

TEA LEAVES	LIQUOR (COLOR)
AROMA	LIQUOR (TASTE)

AROMA CHECK LIST

☐ bitter ☐ robust ☐ nutty ☐ earthy ☐ citrus ☐ flowery ☐ sweet ☐ delicate ☐ malty
☐ spicy ☐ woodsy ☐ smokey ☐ other

PREPARED WITH

☐ sugar ☐ milk ☐ cream ☐ lemon ☐ honey ☐ other

NOTES

IS THIS TEA GOOD ICED?	PURCHASED FROM	
☐ yes ☐ no		
WOULD YOU BUY AGAIN?	IDEAL FOR	RATING
☐ yes ☐ no		☆ ☆ ☆ ☆ ☆

TEA TASTING NOTES

DATE	TEA (NAME/BRAND/SELLER)		
COUNTRY OF ORIGIN:			PRICE

TEA TYPE

☐ black ☐ green ☐ white ☐ herbal ☐ oolong ☐ pu-erh ☐ fruit ☐ other

BREWING METHOD	DRY LEAVES (AMOUNT)	WATER TEMP.	STEEPING TIME(S)

TEA LEAVES	LIQUOR (COLOR)
AROMA	LIQUOR (TASTE)

AROMA CHECK LIST

☐ bitter ☐ robust ☐ nutty ☐ earthy ☐ citrus ☐ flowery ☐ sweet ☐ delicate ☐ malty
☐ spicy ☐ woodsy ☐ smokey ☐ other

PREPARED WITH

☐ sugar ☐ milk ☐ cream ☐ lemon ☐ honey ☐ other

NOTES

IS THIS TEA GOOD ICED? ☐ yes ☐ no	PURCHASED FROM		
WOULD YOU BUY AGAIN? ☐ yes ☐ no	IDEAL FOR		RATING ☆ ☆ ☆ ☆ ☆

TEA TASTING NOTES

DATE	TEA (NAME/BRAND/SELLER)		
COUNTRY OF ORIGIN:			PRICE

TEA TYPE

☐ black   ☐ green   ☐ white   ☐ herbal   ☐ oolong   ☐ pu-erh   ☐ fruit   ☐ other

BREWING METHOD	DRY LEAVES (AMOUNT)	WATER TEMP.	STEEPING TIME(S)

TEA LEAVES	LIQUOR (COLOR)
AROMA	LIQUOR (TASTE)

AROMA CHECK LIST

☐ bitter   ☐ robust   ☐ nutty   ☐ earthy   ☐ citrus   ☐ flowery   ☐ sweet   ☐ delicate   ☐ malty

☐ spicy   ☐ woodsy   ☐ smokey   ☐ other

PREPARED WITH

☐ sugar   ☐ milk   ☐ cream   ☐ lemon   ☐ honey   ☐ other

NOTES

IS THIS TEA GOOD ICED? ☐ yes ☐ no	PURCHASED FROM	
WOULD YOU BUY AGAIN? ☐ yes ☐ no	IDEAL FOR	RATING ☆☆☆☆☆

TEA TASTING NOTES

DATE	TEA (NAME/BRAND/SELLER)

COUNTRY OF ORIGIN:	PRICE

TEA TYPE

☐ black ☐ green ☐ white ☐ herbal ☐ oolong ☐ pu-erh ☐ fruit ☐ other

BREWING METHOD	DRY LEAVES (AMOUNT)	WATER TEMP.	STEEPING TIME(S)

TEA LEAVES	LIQUOR (COLOR)

AROMA	LIQUOR (TASTE)

AROMA CHECK LIST

☐ bitter ☐ robust ☐ nutty ☐ earthy ☐ citrus ☐ flowery ☐ sweet ☐ delicate ☐ malty

☐ spicy ☐ woodsy ☐ smokey ☐ other

PREPARED WITH

☐ sugar ☐ milk ☐ cream ☐ lemon ☐ honey ☐ other

NOTES

IS THIS TEA GOOD ICED?	PURCHASED FROM		
☐ yes ☐ no			
WOULD YOU BUY AGAIN?	IDEAL FOR		RATING
☐ yes ☐ no			☆☆☆☆☆

TEA TASTING NOTES

DATE	TEA (NAME/BRAND/SELLER)	
COUNTRY OF ORIGIN:		PRICE

TEA TYPE

☐ black ☐ green ☐ white ☐ herbal ☐ oolong ☐ pu-erh ☐ fruit ☐ other

BREWING METHOD	DRY LEAVES (AMOUNT)	WATER TEMP.	STEEPING TIME(S)

TEA LEAVES	LIQUOR (COLOR)
AROMA	LIQUOR (TASTE)

AROMA CHECK LIST

☐ bitter ☐ robust ☐ nutty ☐ earthy ☐ citrus ☐ flowery ☐ sweet ☐ delicate ☐ malty
☐ spicy ☐ woodsy ☐ smokey ☐ other

PREPARED WITH

☐ sugar ☐ milk ☐ cream ☐ lemon ☐ honey ☐ other

NOTES

IS THIS TEA GOOD ICED? ☐ yes ☐ no	PURCHASED FROM	
WOULD YOU BUY AGAIN? ☐ yes ☐ no	IDEAL FOR	RATING ☆☆☆☆☆

TEA TASTING NOTES

DATE	TEA (NAME/BRAND/SELLER)	
COUNTRY OF ORIGIN:		PRICE

TEA TYPE

☐ black ☐ green ☐ white ☐ herbal ☐ oolong ☐ pu-erh ☐ fruit ☐ other

BREWING METHOD	DRY LEAVES (AMOUNT)	WATER TEMP.	STEEPING TIME(S)

TEA LEAVES	LIQUOR (COLOR)
AROMA	LIQUOR (TASTE)

AROMA CHECK LIST

☐ bitter ☐ robust ☐ nutty ☐ earthy ☐ citrus ☐ flowery ☐ sweet ☐ delicate ☐ malty

☐ spicy ☐ woodsy ☐ smokey ☐ other

PREPARED WITH

☐ sugar ☐ milk ☐ cream ☐ lemon ☐ honey ☐ other

NOTES

IS THIS TEA GOOD ICED?	PURCHASED FROM	
☐ yes ☐ no		
WOULD YOU BUY AGAIN?	IDEAL FOR	RATING
☐ yes ☐ no		☆☆☆☆☆

TEA TASTING NOTES

DATE	TEA (NAME/BRAND/SELLER)	
COUNTRY OF ORIGIN:		PRICE

TEA TYPE

☐ black   ☐ green   ☐ white   ☐ herbal   ☐ oolong   ☐ pu-erh   ☐ fruit   ☐ other

BREWING METHOD	DRY LEAVES (AMOUNT)	WATER TEMP.	STEEPING TIME(S)

TEA LEAVES	LIQUOR (COLOR)

AROMA	LIQUOR (TASTE)

AROMA CHECK LIST

☐ bitter   ☐ robust   ☐ nutty   ☐ earthy   ☐ citrus   ☐ flowery   ☐ sweet   ☐ delicate   ☐ malty
☐ spicy   ☐ woodsy   ☐ smokey   ☐ other

PREPARED WITH

☐ sugar   ☐ milk   ☐ cream   ☐ lemon   ☐ honey   ☐ other

NOTES

IS THIS TEA GOOD ICED? ☐ yes ☐ no	PURCHASED FROM	
WOULD YOU BUY AGAIN? ☐ yes ☐ no	IDEAL FOR	RATING ☆☆☆☆☆

TEA TASTING NOTES

DATE	TEA (NAME/BRAND/SELLER)	
COUNTRY OF ORIGIN:		PRICE

TEA TYPE

☐ black ☐ green ☐ white ☐ herbal ☐ oolong ☐ pu-erh ☐ fruit ☐ other

BREWING METHOD	DRY LEAVES (AMOUNT)	WATER TEMP.	STEEPING TIME(S)

TEA LEAVES	LIQUOR (COLOR)
AROMA	LIQUOR (TASTE)

AROMA CHECK LIST

☐ bitter ☐ robust ☐ nutty ☐ earthy ☐ citrus ☐ flowery ☐ sweet ☐ delicate ☐ malty
☐ spicy ☐ woodsy ☐ smokey ☐ other

PREPARED WITH

☐ sugar ☐ milk ☐ cream ☐ lemon ☐ honey ☐ other

NOTES

IS THIS TEA GOOD ICED?	PURCHASED FROM	
☐ yes ☐ no		
WOULD YOU BUY AGAIN?	IDEAL FOR	RATING
☐ yes ☐ no		☆☆☆☆☆

TEA TASTING NOTES

DATE	TEA (NAME/BRAND/SELLER)	
COUNTRY OF ORIGIN:		PRICE

TEA TYPE

☐ black ☐ green ☐ white ☐ herbal ☐ oolong ☐ pu-erh ☐ fruit ☐ other

BREWING METHOD	DRY LEAVES (AMOUNT)	WATER TEMP.	STEEPING TIME(S)

TEA LEAVES	LIQUOR (COLOR)
AROMA	LIQUOR (TASTE)

AROMA CHECK LIST

☐ bitter ☐ robust ☐ nutty ☐ earthy ☐ citrus ☐ flowery ☐ sweet ☐ delicate ☐ malty
☐ spicy ☐ woodsy ☐ smokey ☐ other

PREPARED WITH

☐ sugar ☐ milk ☐ cream ☐ lemon ☐ honey ☐ other

NOTES

IS THIS TEA GOOD ICED? ☐ yes ☐ no	PURCHASED FROM	
WOULD YOU BUY AGAIN? ☐ yes ☐ no	IDEAL FOR	RATING ☆☆☆☆☆

TEA TASTING NOTES

DATE	TEA (NAME/BRAND/SELLER)		
COUNTRY OF ORIGIN:			PRICE

TEA TYPE

☐ black ☐ green ☐ white ☐ herbal ☐ oolong ☐ pu-erh ☐ fruit ☐ other

BREWING METHOD	DRY LEAVES (AMOUNT)	WATER TEMP.	STEEPING TIME(S)

TEA LEAVES	LIQUOR (COLOR)
AROMA	LIQUOR (TASTE)

AROMA CHECK LIST

☐ bitter ☐ robust ☐ nutty ☐ earthy ☐ citrus ☐ flowery ☐ sweet ☐ delicate ☐ malty
☐ spicy ☐ woodsy ☐ smokey ☐ other

PREPARED WITH

☐ sugar ☐ milk ☐ cream ☐ lemon ☐ honey ☐ other

NOTES

IS THIS TEA GOOD ICED? ☐ yes ☐ no	PURCHASED FROM		
WOULD YOU BUY AGAIN? ☐ yes ☐ no	IDEAL FOR		RATING ☆ ☆ ☆ ☆ ☆

TEA TASTING NOTES

DATE	TEA (NAME/BRAND/SELLER)	
COUNTRY OF ORIGIN:		PRICE

TEA TYPE

☐ black ☐ green ☐ white ☐ herbal ☐ oolong ☐ pu-erh ☐ fruit ☐ other

BREWING METHOD	DRY LEAVES (AMOUNT)	WATER TEMP.	STEEPING TIME(S)

TEA LEAVES	LIQUOR (COLOR)
AROMA	LIQUOR (TASTE)

AROMA CHECK LIST

☐ bitter ☐ robust ☐ nutty ☐ earthy ☐ citrus ☐ flowery ☐ sweet ☐ delicate ☐ malty
☐ spicy ☐ woodsy ☐ smokey ☐ other

PREPARED WITH

☐ sugar ☐ milk ☐ cream ☐ lemon ☐ honey ☐ other

NOTES

IS THIS TEA GOOD ICED? ☐ yes ☐ no	PURCHASED FROM	
WOULD YOU BUY AGAIN? ☐ yes ☐ no	IDEAL FOR	RATING ☆☆☆☆☆

TEA TASTING NOTES

DATE	TEA (NAME/BRAND/SELLER)	
COUNTRY OF ORIGIN:		PRICE

TEA TYPE

☐ black   ☐ green   ☐ white   ☐ herbal   ☐ oolong   ☐ pu-erh   ☐ fruit   ☐ other

BREWING METHOD	DRY LEAVES (AMOUNT)	WATER TEMP.	STEEPING TIME(S)

TEA LEAVES	LIQUOR (COLOR)
AROMA	LIQUOR (TASTE)

AROMA CHECK LIST

☐ bitter   ☐ robust   ☐ nutty   ☐ earthy   ☐ citrus   ☐ flowery   ☐ sweet   ☐ delicate   ☐ malty

☐ spicy   ☐ woodsy   ☐ smokey   ☐ other

PREPARED WITH

☐ sugar   ☐ milk   ☐ cream   ☐ lemon   ☐ honey   ☐ other

NOTES

IS THIS TEA GOOD ICED?	PURCHASED FROM	
☐ yes ☐ no		
WOULD YOU BUY AGAIN?	IDEAL FOR	RATING
☐ yes ☐ no		☆☆☆☆☆

TEA TASTING NOTES

DATE	TEA (NAME/BRAND/SELLER)	
COUNTRY OF ORIGIN:		PRICE

TEA TYPE

☐ black ☐ green ☐ white ☐ herbal ☐ oolong ☐ pu-erh ☐ fruit ☐ other

BREWING METHOD	DRY LEAVES (AMOUNT)	WATER TEMP.	STEEPING TIME(S)

TEA LEAVES	LIQUOR (COLOR)
AROMA	LIQUOR (TASTE)

AROMA CHECK LIST

☐ bitter ☐ robust ☐ nutty ☐ earthy ☐ citrus ☐ flowery ☐ sweet ☐ delicate ☐ malty
☐ spicy ☐ woodsy ☐ smokey ☐ other

PREPARED WITH

☐ sugar ☐ milk ☐ cream ☐ lemon ☐ honey ☐ other

NOTES

IS THIS TEA GOOD ICED? ☐ yes ☐ no	PURCHASED FROM	
WOULD YOU BUY AGAIN? ☐ yes ☐ no	IDEAL FOR	RATING ☆☆☆☆☆

TEA TASTING NOTES

DATE	TEA (NAME/BRAND/SELLER)	
COUNTRY OF ORIGIN:		PRICE

TEA TYPE

☐ black ☐ green ☐ white ☐ herbal ☐ oolong ☐ pu-erh ☐ fruit ☐ other

BREWING METHOD	DRY LEAVES (AMOUNT)	WATER TEMP.	STEEPING TIME(S)

TEA LEAVES	LIQUOR (COLOR)
AROMA	LIQUOR (TASTE)

AROMA CHECK LIST

☐ bitter ☐ robust ☐ nutty ☐ earthy ☐ citrus ☐ flowery ☐ sweet ☐ delicate ☐ malty
☐ spicy ☐ woodsy ☐ smokey ☐ other

PREPARED WITH

☐ sugar ☐ milk ☐ cream ☐ lemon ☐ honey ☐ other

NOTES

IS THIS TEA GOOD ICED?	PURCHASED FROM	
☐ yes ☐ no		
WOULD YOU BUY AGAIN?	IDEAL FOR	RATING
☐ yes ☐ no		☆☆☆☆☆

TEA TASTING NOTES

DATE	TEA (NAME/BRAND/SELLER)	
COUNTRY OF ORIGIN:		PRICE

TEA TYPE

☐ black ☐ green ☐ white ☐ herbal ☐ oolong ☐ pu-erh ☐ fruit ☐ other

BREWING METHOD	DRY LEAVES (AMOUNT)	WATER TEMP.	STEEPING TIME(S)

TEA LEAVES	LIQUOR (COLOR)
AROMA	LIQUOR (TASTE)

AROMA CHECK LIST

☐ bitter ☐ robust ☐ nutty ☐ earthy ☐ citrus ☐ flowery ☐ sweet ☐ delicate ☐ malty
☐ spicy ☐ woodsy ☐ smokey ☐ other

PREPARED WITH

☐ sugar ☐ milk ☐ cream ☐ lemon ☐ honey ☐ other

NOTES

IS THIS TEA GOOD ICED?	PURCHASED FROM	
☐ yes ☐ no		
WOULD YOU BUY AGAIN?	IDEAL FOR	RATING
☐ yes ☐ no		☆☆☆☆☆

TEA TASTING NOTES

DATE	TEA (NAME/BRAND/SELLER)	
COUNTRY OF ORIGIN:		PRICE

TEA TYPE

☐ black   ☐ green   ☐ white   ☐ herbal   ☐ oolong   ☐ pu-erh   ☐ fruit   ☐ other

BREWING METHOD	DRY LEAVES (AMOUNT)	WATER TEMP.	STEEPING TIME(S)

TEA LEAVES	LIQUOR (COLOR)
AROMA	LIQUOR (TASTE)

AROMA CHECK LIST

☐ bitter   ☐ robust   ☐ nutty   ☐ earthy   ☐ citrus   ☐ flowery   ☐ sweet   ☐ delicate   ☐ malty

☐ spicy   ☐ woodsy   ☐ smokey   ☐ other

PREPARED WITH

☐ sugar   ☐ milk   ☐ cream   ☐ lemon   ☐ honey   ☐ other

NOTES

IS THIS TEA GOOD ICED?	PURCHASED FROM	
☐ yes ☐ no		
WOULD YOU BUY AGAIN?	IDEAL FOR	RATING
☐ yes ☐ no		☆ ☆ ☆ ☆ ☆

TEA TASTING NOTES

DATE	TEA (NAME/BRAND/SELLER)	
COUNTRY OF ORIGIN:		PRICE

TEA TYPE

☐ black ☐ green ☐ white ☐ herbal ☐ oolong ☐ pu-erh ☐ fruit ☐ other

BREWING METHOD	DRY LEAVES (AMOUNT)	WATER TEMP.	STEEPING TIME(S)

TEA LEAVES	LIQUOR (COLOR)
AROMA	LIQUOR (TASTE)

AROMA CHECK LIST

☐ bitter ☐ robust ☐ nutty ☐ earthy ☐ citrus ☐ flowery ☐ sweet ☐ delicate ☐ malty
☐ spicy ☐ woodsy ☐ smokey ☐ other

PREPARED WITH

☐ sugar ☐ milk ☐ cream ☐ lemon ☐ honey ☐ other

NOTES

IS THIS TEA GOOD ICED? ☐ yes ☐ no	PURCHASED FROM	
WOULD YOU BUY AGAIN? ☐ yes ☐ no	IDEAL FOR	RATING ☆☆☆☆☆

TEA TASTING NOTES

DATE	TEA (NAME/BRAND/SELLER)	
COUNTRY OF ORIGIN:		PRICE

TEA TYPE

☐ black ☐ green ☐ white ☐ herbal ☐ oolong ☐ pu-erh ☐ fruit ☐ other

BREWING METHOD	DRY LEAVES (AMOUNT)	WATER TEMP.	STEEPING TIME(S)

TEA LEAVES	LIQUOR (COLOR)

AROMA	LIQUOR (TASTE)

AROMA CHECK LIST

☐ bitter ☐ robust ☐ nutty ☐ earthy ☐ citrus ☐ flowery ☐ sweet ☐ delicate ☐ malty
☐ spicy ☐ woodsy ☐ smokey ☐ other

PREPARED WITH

☐ sugar ☐ milk ☐ cream ☐ lemon ☐ honey ☐ other

NOTES

IS THIS TEA GOOD ICED?	PURCHASED FROM	
☐ yes ☐ no		
WOULD YOU BUY AGAIN?	IDEAL FOR	RATING
☐ yes ☐ no		☆ ☆ ☆ ☆ ☆

TEA TASTING NOTES

DATE	TEA (NAME/BRAND/SELLER)	
COUNTRY OF ORIGIN:		PRICE

TEA TYPE

☐ black ☐ green ☐ white ☐ herbal ☐ oolong ☐ pu-erh ☐ fruit ☐ other

BREWING METHOD	DRY LEAVES (AMOUNT)	WATER TEMP.	STEEPING TIME(S)

TEA LEAVES	LIQUOR (COLOR)
AROMA	LIQUOR (TASTE)

AROMA CHECK LIST

☐ bitter ☐ robust ☐ nutty ☐ earthy ☐ citrus ☐ flowery ☐ sweet ☐ delicate ☐ malty
☐ spicy ☐ woodsy ☐ smokey ☐ other

PREPARED WITH

☐ sugar ☐ milk ☐ cream ☐ lemon ☐ honey ☐ other

NOTES

IS THIS TEA GOOD ICED?	PURCHASED FROM	
☐ yes ☐ no		
WOULD YOU BUY AGAIN?	IDEAL FOR	RATING
☐ yes ☐ no		☆☆☆☆☆

TEA TASTING NOTES

DATE	TEA (NAME/BRAND/SELLER)	
COUNTRY OF ORIGIN:		PRICE

TEA TYPE

☐ black ☐ green ☐ white ☐ herbal ☐ oolong ☐ pu-erh ☐ fruit ☐ other

BREWING METHOD	DRY LEAVES (AMOUNT)	WATER TEMP.	STEEPING TIME(S)

TEA LEAVES	LIQUOR (COLOR)

AROMA	LIQUOR (TASTE)

AROMA CHECK LIST

☐ bitter ☐ robust ☐ nutty ☐ earthy ☐ citrus ☐ flowery ☐ sweet ☐ delicate ☐ malty
☐ spicy ☐ woodsy ☐ smokey ☐ other

PREPARED WITH

☐ sugar ☐ milk ☐ cream ☐ lemon ☐ honey ☐ other

NOTES

IS THIS TEA GOOD ICED? ☐ yes ☐ no	PURCHASED FROM	
WOULD YOU BUY AGAIN? ☐ yes ☐ no	IDEAL FOR	RATING ☆☆☆☆☆

TEA TASTING NOTES

DATE	TEA (NAME/BRAND/SELLER)	
COUNTRY OF ORIGIN:		PRICE

TEA TYPE

☐ black ☐ green ☐ white ☐ herbal ☐ oolong ☐ pu-erh ☐ fruit ☐ other

BREWING METHOD	DRY LEAVES (AMOUNT)	WATER TEMP.	STEEPING TIME(S)

TEA LEAVES	LIQUOR (COLOR)
AROMA	LIQUOR (TASTE)

AROMA CHECK LIST

☐ bitter ☐ robust ☐ nutty ☐ earthy ☐ citrus ☐ flowery ☐ sweet ☐ delicate ☐ malty
☐ spicy ☐ woodsy ☐ smokey ☐ other

PREPARED WITH

☐ sugar ☐ milk ☐ cream ☐ lemon ☐ honey ☐ other

NOTES

IS THIS TEA GOOD ICED?	PURCHASED FROM	
☐ yes ☐ no		
WOULD YOU BUY AGAIN?	IDEAL FOR	RATING
☐ yes ☐ no		☆ ☆ ☆ ☆ ☆

TEA TASTING NOTES

DATE	TEA (NAME/BRAND/SELLER)	
COUNTRY OF ORIGIN:		PRICE

TEA TYPE

☐ black ☐ green ☐ white ☐ herbal ☐ oolong ☐ pu-erh ☐ fruit ☐ other

BREWING METHOD	DRY LEAVES (AMOUNT)	WATER TEMP.	STEEPING TIME(S)

TEA LEAVES	LIQUOR (COLOR)
AROMA	LIQUOR (TASTE)

AROMA CHECK LIST

☐ bitter ☐ robust ☐ nutty ☐ earthy ☐ citrus ☐ flowery ☐ sweet ☐ delicate ☐ malty
☐ spicy ☐ woodsy ☐ smokey ☐ other

PREPARED WITH

☐ sugar ☐ milk ☐ cream ☐ lemon ☐ honey ☐ other

NOTES

IS THIS TEA GOOD ICED? ☐ yes ☐ no	PURCHASED FROM	
WOULD YOU BUY AGAIN? ☐ yes ☐ no	IDEAL FOR	RATING ☆ ☆ ☆ ☆ ☆

TEA TASTING NOTES

DATE	TEA (NAME/BRAND/SELLER)	
COUNTRY OF ORIGIN:		PRICE

TEA TYPE

☐ black ☐ green ☐ white ☐ herbal ☐ oolong ☐ pu-erh ☐ fruit ☐ other

BREWING METHOD	DRY LEAVES (AMOUNT)	WATER TEMP.	STEEPING TIME(S)

TEA LEAVES	LIQUOR (COLOR)
AROMA	LIQUOR (TASTE)

AROMA CHECK LIST

☐ bitter ☐ robust ☐ nutty ☐ earthy ☐ citrus ☐ flowery ☐ sweet ☐ delicate ☐ malty

☐ spicy ☐ woodsy ☐ smokey ☐ other

PREPARED WITH

☐ sugar ☐ milk ☐ cream ☐ lemon ☐ honey ☐ other

NOTES

IS THIS TEA GOOD ICED?	PURCHASED FROM	
☐ yes ☐ no		
WOULD YOU BUY AGAIN?	IDEAL FOR	RATING
☐ yes ☐ no		☆☆☆☆☆

TEA TASTING NOTES

DATE	TEA (NAME/BRAND/SELLER)	
COUNTRY OF ORIGIN:		PRICE

TEA TYPE
☐ black ☐ green ☐ white ☐ herbal ☐ oolong ☐ pu-erh ☐ fruit ☐ other

BREWING METHOD	DRY LEAVES (AMOUNT)	WATER TEMP.	STEEPING TIME(S)

TEA LEAVES	LIQUOR (COLOR)
AROMA	LIQUOR (TASTE)

AROMA CHECK LIST
☐ bitter ☐ robust ☐ nutty ☐ earthy ☐ citrus ☐ flowery ☐ sweet ☐ delicate ☐ malty
☐ spicy ☐ woodsy ☐ smokey ☐ other

PREPARED WITH
☐ sugar ☐ milk ☐ cream ☐ lemon ☐ honey ☐ other

NOTES

IS THIS TEA GOOD ICED?	PURCHASED FROM	
☐ yes ☐ no		
WOULD YOU BUY AGAIN?	IDEAL FOR	RATING
☐ yes ☐ no		☆☆☆☆☆

TEA TASTING NOTES

DATE	TEA (NAME/BRAND/SELLER)	
COUNTRY OF ORIGIN:		PRICE

TEA TYPE

☐ black ☐ green ☐ white ☐ herbal ☐ oolong ☐ pu-erh ☐ fruit ☐ other

BREWING METHOD	DRY LEAVES (AMOUNT)	WATER TEMP.	STEEPING TIME(S)

TEA LEAVES	LIQUOR (COLOR)
AROMA	LIQUOR (TASTE)

AROMA CHECK LIST

☐ bitter ☐ robust ☐ nutty ☐ earthy ☐ citrus ☐ flowery ☐ sweet ☐ delicate ☐ malty
☐ spicy ☐ woodsy ☐ smokey ☐ other

PREPARED WITH

☐ sugar ☐ milk ☐ cream ☐ lemon ☐ honey ☐ other

NOTES

IS THIS TEA GOOD ICED? ☐ yes ☐ no	PURCHASED FROM	
WOULD YOU BUY AGAIN? ☐ yes ☐ no	IDEAL FOR	RATING ☆☆☆☆☆

TEA TASTING NOTES

DATE	TEA (NAME/BRAND/SELLER)	
COUNTRY OF ORIGIN:		PRICE

TEA TYPE

☐ black ☐ green ☐ white ☐ herbal ☐ oolong ☐ pu-erh ☐ fruit ☐ other

BREWING METHOD	DRY LEAVES (AMOUNT)	WATER TEMP.	STEEPING TIME(S)

TEA LEAVES	LIQUOR (COLOR)
AROMA	LIQUOR (TASTE)

AROMA CHECK LIST

☐ bitter ☐ robust ☐ nutty ☐ earthy ☐ citrus ☐ flowery ☐ sweet ☐ delicate ☐ malty
☐ spicy ☐ woodsy ☐ smokey ☐ other

PREPARED WITH

☐ sugar ☐ milk ☐ cream ☐ lemon ☐ honey ☐ other

NOTES

IS THIS TEA GOOD ICED? ☐ yes ☐ no	PURCHASED FROM	
WOULD YOU BUY AGAIN? ☐ yes ☐ no	IDEAL FOR	RATING ☆ ☆ ☆ ☆ ☆

TEA TASTING NOTES

DATE	TEA (NAME/BRAND/SELLER)	
COUNTRY OF ORIGIN:		PRICE

TEA TYPE

☐ black ☐ green ☐ white ☐ herbal ☐ oolong ☐ pu-erh ☐ fruit ☐ other

BREWING METHOD	DRY LEAVES (AMOUNT)	WATER TEMP.	STEEPING TIME(S)

TEA LEAVES	LIQUOR (COLOR)
AROMA	LIQUOR (TASTE)

AROMA CHECK LIST

☐ bitter ☐ robust ☐ nutty ☐ earthy ☐ citrus ☐ flowery ☐ sweet ☐ delicate ☐ malty

☐ spicy ☐ woodsy ☐ smokey ☐ other

PREPARED WITH

☐ sugar ☐ milk ☐ cream ☐ lemon ☐ honey ☐ other

NOTES

IS THIS TEA GOOD ICED?	PURCHASED FROM	
☐ yes ☐ no		
WOULD YOU BUY AGAIN?	IDEAL FOR	RATING
☐ yes ☐ no		☆☆☆☆☆

TEA TASTING NOTES

DATE	TEA (NAME/BRAND/SELLER)	
COUNTRY OF ORIGIN:		PRICE

TEA TYPE

☐ black ☐ green ☐ white ☐ herbal ☐ oolong ☐ pu-erh ☐ fruit ☐ other

BREWING METHOD	DRY LEAVES (AMOUNT)	WATER TEMP.	STEEPING TIME(S)

TEA LEAVES	LIQUOR (COLOR)
AROMA	LIQUOR (TASTE)

AROMA CHECK LIST

☐ bitter ☐ robust ☐ nutty ☐ earthy ☐ citrus ☐ flowery ☐ sweet ☐ delicate ☐ malty

☐ spicy ☐ woodsy ☐ smokey ☐ other

PREPARED WITH

☐ sugar ☐ milk ☐ cream ☐ lemon ☐ honey ☐ other

NOTES

IS THIS TEA GOOD ICED? ☐ yes ☐ no	PURCHASED FROM	
WOULD YOU BUY AGAIN? ☐ yes ☐ no	IDEAL FOR	RATING ☆☆☆☆☆

TEA TASTING NOTES

DATE	TEA (NAME/BRAND/SELLER)	
COUNTRY OF ORIGIN:		PRICE

TEA TYPE

☐ black   ☐ green   ☐ white   ☐ herbal   ☐ oolong   ☐ pu-erh   ☐ fruit   ☐ other

BREWING METHOD	DRY LEAVES (AMOUNT)	WATER TEMP.	STEEPING TIME(S)

TEA LEAVES	LIQUOR (COLOR)
AROMA	LIQUOR (TASTE)

AROMA CHECK LIST

☐ bitter   ☐ robust   ☐ nutty   ☐ earthy   ☐ citrus   ☐ flowery   ☐ sweet   ☐ delicate   ☐ malty

☐ spicy   ☐ woodsy   ☐ smokey   ☐ other

PREPARED WITH

☐ sugar   ☐ milk   ☐ cream   ☐ lemon   ☐ honey   ☐ other

NOTES

IS THIS TEA GOOD ICED?	PURCHASED FROM	
☐ yes ☐ no		
WOULD YOU BUY AGAIN?	IDEAL FOR	RATING
☐ yes ☐ no		☆☆☆☆☆

TEA TASTING NOTES

DATE	TEA (NAME/BRAND/SELLER)	
COUNTRY OF ORIGIN:		PRICE

TEA TYPE

☐ black ☐ green ☐ white ☐ herbal ☐ oolong ☐ pu-erh ☐ fruit ☐ other

BREWING METHOD	DRY LEAVES (AMOUNT)	WATER TEMP.	STEEPING TIME(S)

TEA LEAVES	LIQUOR (COLOR)
AROMA	LIQUOR (TASTE)

AROMA CHECK LIST

☐ bitter ☐ robust ☐ nutty ☐ earthy ☐ citrus ☐ flowery ☐ sweet ☐ delicate ☐ malty
☐ spicy ☐ woodsy ☐ smokey ☐ other

PREPARED WITH

☐ sugar ☐ milk ☐ cream ☐ lemon ☐ honey ☐ other

NOTES

IS THIS TEA GOOD ICED?	PURCHASED FROM	
☐ yes ☐ no		
WOULD YOU BUY AGAIN?	IDEAL FOR	RATING
☐ yes ☐ no		☆☆☆☆☆

TEA TASTING NOTES

DATE	TEA (NAME/BRAND/SELLER)	
COUNTRY OF ORIGIN:		PRICE

TEA TYPE

☐ black ☐ green ☐ white ☐ herbal ☐ oolong ☐ pu-erh ☐ fruit ☐ other

BREWING METHOD	DRY LEAVES (AMOUNT)	WATER TEMP.	STEEPING TIME(S)

TEA LEAVES	LIQUOR (COLOR)
AROMA	LIQUOR (TASTE)

AROMA CHECK LIST

☐ bitter ☐ robust ☐ nutty ☐ earthy ☐ citrus ☐ flowery ☐ sweet ☐ delicate ☐ malty

☐ spicy ☐ woodsy ☐ smokey ☐ other

PREPARED WITH

☐ sugar ☐ milk ☐ cream ☐ lemon ☐ honey ☐ other

NOTES

IS THIS TEA GOOD ICED?	PURCHASED FROM	
☐ yes ☐ no		
WOULD YOU BUY AGAIN?	IDEAL FOR	RATING
☐ yes ☐ no		☆☆☆☆☆

TEA TASTING NOTES

DATE	TEA (NAME/BRAND/SELLER)	
COUNTRY OF ORIGIN:		PRICE

TEA TYPE

☐ black ☐ green ☐ white ☐ herbal ☐ oolong ☐ pu-erh ☐ fruit ☐ other

BREWING METHOD	DRY LEAVES (AMOUNT)	WATER TEMP.	STEEPING TIME(S)

TEA LEAVES	LIQUOR (COLOR)
AROMA	LIQUOR (TASTE)

AROMA CHECK LIST

☐ bitter ☐ robust ☐ nutty ☐ earthy ☐ citrus ☐ flowery ☐ sweet ☐ delicate ☐ malty
☐ spicy ☐ woodsy ☐ smokey ☐ other

PREPARED WITH

☐ sugar ☐ milk ☐ cream ☐ lemon ☐ honey ☐ other

NOTES

IS THIS TEA GOOD ICED?	PURCHASED FROM	
☐ yes ☐ no		
WOULD YOU BUY AGAIN?	IDEAL FOR	RATING
☐ yes ☐ no		☆☆☆☆☆

TEA TASTING NOTES

DATE	TEA (NAME/BRAND/SELLER)	
COUNTRY OF ORIGIN:		PRICE

TEA TYPE
☐ black ☐ green ☐ white ☐ herbal ☐ oolong ☐ pu-erh ☐ fruit ☐ other

BREWING METHOD	DRY LEAVES (AMOUNT)	WATER TEMP.	STEEPING TIME(S)

TEA LEAVES	LIQUOR (COLOR)
AROMA	LIQUOR (TASTE)

AROMA CHECK LIST
☐ bitter ☐ robust ☐ nutty ☐ earthy ☐ citrus ☐ flowery ☐ sweet ☐ delicate ☐ malty
☐ spicy ☐ woodsy ☐ smokey ☐ other

PREPARED WITH
☐ sugar ☐ milk ☐ cream ☐ lemon ☐ honey ☐ other

NOTES

IS THIS TEA GOOD ICED? ☐ yes ☐ no	PURCHASED FROM	
WOULD YOU BUY AGAIN? ☐ yes ☐ no	IDEAL FOR	RATING ☆☆☆☆☆

TEA TASTING NOTES

DATE	TEA (NAME/BRAND/SELLER)	
COUNTRY OF ORIGIN:		PRICE

TEA TYPE
☐ black ☐ green ☐ white ☐ herbal ☐ oolong ☐ pu-erh ☐ fruit ☐ other

BREWING METHOD	DRY LEAVES (AMOUNT)	WATER TEMP.	STEEPING TIME(S)

TEA LEAVES	LIQUOR (COLOR)
AROMA	LIQUOR (TASTE)

AROMA CHECK LIST
☐ bitter ☐ robust ☐ nutty ☐ earthy ☐ citrus ☐ flowery ☐ sweet ☐ delicate ☐ malty
☐ spicy ☐ woodsy ☐ smokey ☐ other

PREPARED WITH
☐ sugar ☐ milk ☐ cream ☐ lemon ☐ honey ☐ other

NOTES

IS THIS TEA GOOD ICED? ☐ yes ☐ no	PURCHASED FROM	
WOULD YOU BUY AGAIN? ☐ yes ☐ no	IDEAL FOR	RATING ☆ ☆ ☆ ☆ ☆

TEA TASTING NOTES

DATE	TEA (NAME/BRAND/SELLER)	
COUNTRY OF ORIGIN:		PRICE

TEA TYPE
☐ black ☐ green ☐ white ☐ herbal ☐ oolong ☐ pu-erh ☐ fruit ☐ other

BREWING METHOD	DRY LEAVES (AMOUNT)	WATER TEMP.	STEEPING TIME(S)

TEA LEAVES	LIQUOR (COLOR)
AROMA	LIQUOR (TASTE)

AROMA CHECK LIST
☐ bitter ☐ robust ☐ nutty ☐ earthy ☐ citrus ☐ flowery ☐ sweet ☐ delicate ☐ malty
☐ spicy ☐ woodsy ☐ smokey ☐ other

PREPARED WITH
☐ sugar ☐ milk ☐ cream ☐ lemon ☐ honey ☐ other

NOTES

IS THIS TEA GOOD ICED? ☐ yes ☐ no	PURCHASED FROM	
WOULD YOU BUY AGAIN? ☐ yes ☐ no	IDEAL FOR	RATING ☆☆☆☆☆

TEA TASTING NOTES

DATE	TEA (NAME/BRAND/SELLER)	
COUNTRY OF ORIGIN:		PRICE

TEA TYPE

☐ black ☐ green ☐ white ☐ herbal ☐ oolong ☐ pu-erh ☐ fruit ☐ other

BREWING METHOD	DRY LEAVES (AMOUNT)	WATER TEMP.	STEEPING TIME(S)

TEA LEAVES	LIQUOR (COLOR)
AROMA	LIQUOR (TASTE)

AROMA CHECK LIST

☐ bitter ☐ robust ☐ nutty ☐ earthy ☐ citrus ☐ flowery ☐ sweet ☐ delicate ☐ malty
☐ spicy ☐ woodsy ☐ smokey ☐ other

PREPARED WITH

☐ sugar ☐ milk ☐ cream ☐ lemon ☐ honey ☐ other

NOTES

IS THIS TEA GOOD ICED? ☐ yes ☐ no	PURCHASED FROM	
WOULD YOU BUY AGAIN? ☐ yes ☐ no	IDEAL FOR	RATING ☆ ☆ ☆ ☆ ☆

TEA TASTING NOTES

DATE	TEA (NAME/BRAND/SELLER)	
COUNTRY OF ORIGIN:		PRICE

TEA TYPE

☐ black ☐ green ☐ white ☐ herbal ☐ oolong ☐ pu-erh ☐ fruit ☐ other

BREWING METHOD	DRY LEAVES (AMOUNT)	WATER TEMP.	STEEPING TIME(S)

TEA LEAVES	LIQUOR (COLOR)
AROMA	LIQUOR (TASTE)

AROMA CHECK LIST

☐ bitter ☐ robust ☐ nutty ☐ earthy ☐ citrus ☐ flowery ☐ sweet ☐ delicate ☐ malty
☐ spicy ☐ woodsy ☐ smokey ☐ other

PREPARED WITH

☐ sugar ☐ milk ☐ cream ☐ lemon ☐ honey ☐ other

NOTES

| IS THIS TEA GOOD ICED? ☐ yes ☐ no | PURCHASED FROM | |
| WOULD YOU BUY AGAIN? ☐ yes ☐ no | IDEAL FOR | RATING ☆☆☆☆☆ |

TEA TASTING NOTES

DATE	TEA (NAME/BRAND/SELLER)		
COUNTRY OF ORIGIN:			PRICE

TEA TYPE

☐ black ☐ green ☐ white ☐ herbal ☐ oolong ☐ pu-erh ☐ fruit ☐ other

BREWING METHOD	DRY LEAVES (AMOUNT)	WATER TEMP.	STEEPING TIME(S)

TEA LEAVES	LIQUOR (COLOR)
AROMA	LIQUOR (TASTE)

AROMA CHECK LIST

☐ bitter ☐ robust ☐ nutty ☐ earthy ☐ citrus ☐ flowery ☐ sweet ☐ delicate ☐ malty

☐ spicy ☐ woodsy ☐ smokey ☐ other

PREPARED WITH

☐ sugar ☐ milk ☐ cream ☐ lemon ☐ honey ☐ other

NOTES

IS THIS TEA GOOD ICED? ☐ yes ☐ no	PURCHASED FROM		
WOULD YOU BUY AGAIN? ☐ yes ☐ no	IDEAL FOR		RATING ☆☆☆☆☆

TEA TASTING NOTES

DATE	TEA (NAME/BRAND/SELLER)	
COUNTRY OF ORIGIN:		PRICE

TEA TYPE

☐ black ☐ green ☐ white ☐ herbal ☐ oolong ☐ pu-erh ☐ fruit ☐ other

BREWING METHOD	DRY LEAVES (AMOUNT)	WATER TEMP.	STEEPING TIME(S)

TEA LEAVES	LIQUOR (COLOR)
AROMA	LIQUOR (TASTE)

AROMA CHECK LIST

☐ bitter ☐ robust ☐ nutty ☐ earthy ☐ citrus ☐ flowery ☐ sweet ☐ delicate ☐ malty

☐ spicy ☐ woodsy ☐ smokey ☐ other

PREPARED WITH

☐ sugar ☐ milk ☐ cream ☐ lemon ☐ honey ☐ other

NOTES

IS THIS TEA GOOD ICED?	PURCHASED FROM	
☐ yes ☐ no		
WOULD YOU BUY AGAIN?	IDEAL FOR	RATING
☐ yes ☐ no		☆ ☆ ☆ ☆ ☆

TEA TASTING NOTES

DATE	TEA (NAME/BRAND/SELLER)	
COUNTRY OF ORIGIN:		PRICE

TEA TYPE

☐ black ☐ green ☐ white ☐ herbal ☐ oolong ☐ pu-erh ☐ fruit ☐ other

BREWING METHOD	DRY LEAVES (AMOUNT)	WATER TEMP.	STEEPING TIME(S)

TEA LEAVES	LIQUOR (COLOR)
AROMA	LIQUOR (TASTE)

AROMA CHECK LIST

☐ bitter ☐ robust ☐ nutty ☐ earthy ☐ citrus ☐ flowery ☐ sweet ☐ delicate ☐ malty

☐ spicy ☐ woodsy ☐ smokey ☐ other

PREPARED WITH

☐ sugar ☐ milk ☐ cream ☐ lemon ☐ honey ☐ other

NOTES

IS THIS TEA GOOD ICED?	PURCHASED FROM	
☐ yes ☐ no		
WOULD YOU BUY AGAIN?	IDEAL FOR	RATING
☐ yes ☐ no		☆☆☆☆☆

TEA TASTING NOTES

DATE	TEA (NAME/BRAND/SELLER)	
COUNTRY OF ORIGIN:		PRICE

TEA TYPE

☐ black   ☐ green   ☐ white   ☐ herbal   ☐ oolong   ☐ pu-erh   ☐ fruit   ☐ other

BREWING METHOD	DRY LEAVES (AMOUNT)	WATER TEMP.	STEEPING TIME(S)

TEA LEAVES	LIQUOR (COLOR)
AROMA	LIQUOR (TASTE)

AROMA CHECK LIST

☐ bitter   ☐ robust   ☐ nutty   ☐ earthy   ☐ citrus   ☐ flowery   ☐ sweet   ☐ delicate   ☐ malty

☐ spicy   ☐ woodsy   ☐ smokey   ☐ other

PREPARED WITH

☐ sugar   ☐ milk   ☐ cream   ☐ lemon   ☐ honey   ☐ other

NOTES

IS THIS TEA GOOD ICED?	PURCHASED FROM	
☐ yes ☐ no		
WOULD YOU BUY AGAIN?	IDEAL FOR	RATING
☐ yes ☐ no		☆ ☆ ☆ ☆ ☆

TEA TASTING NOTES

DATE	TEA (NAME/BRAND/SELLER)	
COUNTRY OF ORIGIN:		PRICE

TEA TYPE

☐ black ☐ green ☐ white ☐ herbal ☐ oolong ☐ pu-erh ☐ fruit ☐ other

BREWING METHOD	DRY LEAVES (AMOUNT)	WATER TEMP.	STEEPING TIME(S)

TEA LEAVES	LIQUOR (COLOR)
AROMA	LIQUOR (TASTE)

AROMA CHECK LIST

☐ bitter ☐ robust ☐ nutty ☐ earthy ☐ citrus ☐ flowery ☐ sweet ☐ delicate ☐ malty
☐ spicy ☐ woodsy ☐ smokey ☐ other

PREPARED WITH

☐ sugar ☐ milk ☐ cream ☐ lemon ☐ honey ☐ other

NOTES

IS THIS TEA GOOD ICED? ☐ yes ☐ no	PURCHASED FROM	
WOULD YOU BUY AGAIN? ☐ yes ☐ no	IDEAL FOR	RATING ☆☆☆☆☆

TEA TASTING NOTES

DATE	TEA (NAME/BRAND/SELLER)	
COUNTRY OF ORIGIN:		PRICE

TEA TYPE
☐ black ☐ green ☐ white ☐ herbal ☐ oolong ☐ pu-erh ☐ fruit ☐ other

BREWING METHOD	DRY LEAVES (AMOUNT)	WATER TEMP.	STEEPING TIME(S)

TEA LEAVES	LIQUOR (COLOR)
AROMA	LIQUOR (TASTE)

AROMA CHECK LIST
☐ bitter ☐ robust ☐ nutty ☐ earthy ☐ citrus ☐ flowery ☐ sweet ☐ delicate ☐ malty
☐ spicy ☐ woodsy ☐ smokey ☐ other

PREPARED WITH
☐ sugar ☐ milk ☐ cream ☐ lemon ☐ honey ☐ other

NOTES

IS THIS TEA GOOD ICED?	PURCHASED FROM
☐ yes ☐ no	

WOULD YOU BUY AGAIN?	IDEAL FOR	RATING
☐ yes ☐ no		☆ ☆ ☆ ☆ ☆

TEA TASTING NOTES

DATE	TEA (NAME/BRAND/SELLER)		
COUNTRY OF ORIGIN:			PRICE

TEA TYPE

☐ black ☐ green ☐ white ☐ herbal ☐ oolong ☐ pu-erh ☐ fruit ☐ other

BREWING METHOD	DRY LEAVES (AMOUNT)	WATER TEMP.	STEEPING TIME(S)

TEA LEAVES	LIQUOR (COLOR)
AROMA	LIQUOR (TASTE)

AROMA CHECK LIST

☐ bitter ☐ robust ☐ nutty ☐ earthy ☐ citrus ☐ flowery ☐ sweet ☐ delicate ☐ malty
☐ spicy ☐ woodsy ☐ smokey ☐ other

PREPARED WITH

☐ sugar ☐ milk ☐ cream ☐ lemon ☐ honey ☐ other

NOTES

IS THIS TEA GOOD ICED? ☐ yes ☐ no	PURCHASED FROM		
WOULD YOU BUY AGAIN? ☐ yes ☐ no	IDEAL FOR		RATING ☆ ☆ ☆ ☆ ☆

TEA TASTING NOTES

DATE	TEA (NAME/BRAND/SELLER)		
COUNTRY OF ORIGIN:			PRICE

TEA TYPE

☐ black ☐ green ☐ white ☐ herbal ☐ oolong ☐ pu-erh ☐ fruit ☐ other

BREWING METHOD	DRY LEAVES (AMOUNT)	WATER TEMP.	STEEPING TIME(S)

TEA LEAVES	LIQUOR (COLOR)
AROMA	LIQUOR (TASTE)

AROMA CHECK LIST

☐ bitter ☐ robust ☐ nutty ☐ earthy ☐ citrus ☐ flowery ☐ sweet ☐ delicate ☐ malty

☐ spicy ☐ woodsy ☐ smokey ☐ other

PREPARED WITH

☐ sugar ☐ milk ☐ cream ☐ lemon ☐ honey ☐ other

NOTES

IS THIS TEA GOOD ICED?	PURCHASED FROM		
☐ yes ☐ no			
WOULD YOU BUY AGAIN?	IDEAL FOR		RATING
☐ yes ☐ no			☆ ☆ ☆ ☆ ☆

TEA TASTING NOTES

DATE	TEA (NAME/BRAND/SELLER)	
COUNTRY OF ORIGIN:		PRICE

TEA TYPE

☐ black ☐ green ☐ white ☐ herbal ☐ oolong ☐ pu-erh ☐ fruit ☐ other

BREWING METHOD	DRY LEAVES (AMOUNT)	WATER TEMP.	STEEPING TIME(S)

TEA LEAVES	LIQUOR (COLOR)

AROMA	LIQUOR (TASTE)

AROMA CHECK LIST

☐ bitter ☐ robust ☐ nutty ☐ earthy ☐ citrus ☐ flowery ☐ sweet ☐ delicate ☐ malty
☐ spicy ☐ woodsy ☐ smokey ☐ other

PREPARED WITH

☐ sugar ☐ milk ☐ cream ☐ lemon ☐ honey ☐ other

NOTES

IS THIS TEA GOOD ICED?	PURCHASED FROM	
☐ yes ☐ no		
WOULD YOU BUY AGAIN?	IDEAL FOR	RATING
☐ yes ☐ no		☆ ☆ ☆ ☆ ☆

TEA TASTING NOTES

DATE	TEA (NAME/BRAND/SELLER)	
COUNTRY OF ORIGIN:		PRICE

TEA TYPE
☐ black ☐ green ☐ white ☐ herbal ☐ oolong ☐ pu-erh ☐ fruit ☐ other

BREWING METHOD	DRY LEAVES (AMOUNT)	WATER TEMP.	STEEPING TIME(S)

TEA LEAVES	LIQUOR (COLOR)
AROMA	LIQUOR (TASTE)

AROMA CHECK LIST
☐ bitter ☐ robust ☐ nutty ☐ earthy ☐ citrus ☐ flowery ☐ sweet ☐ delicate ☐ malty
☐ spicy ☐ woodsy ☐ smokey ☐ other

PREPARED WITH
☐ sugar ☐ milk ☐ cream ☐ lemon ☐ honey ☐ other

NOTES

IS THIS TEA GOOD ICED?	PURCHASED FROM	
☐ yes ☐ no		
WOULD YOU BUY AGAIN?	IDEAL FOR	RATING
☐ yes ☐ no		☆ ☆ ☆ ☆ ☆

TEA TASTING NOTES

DATE	TEA (NAME/BRAND/SELLER)		
COUNTRY OF ORIGIN:			PRICE

TEA TYPE

☐ black ☐ green ☐ white ☐ herbal ☐ oolong ☐ pu-erh ☐ fruit ☐ other

BREWING METHOD	DRY LEAVES (AMOUNT)	WATER TEMP.	STEEPING TIME(S)

TEA LEAVES	LIQUOR (COLOR)
AROMA	LIQUOR (TASTE)

AROMA CHECK LIST

☐ bitter ☐ robust ☐ nutty ☐ earthy ☐ citrus ☐ flowery ☐ sweet ☐ delicate ☐ malty
☐ spicy ☐ woodsy ☐ smokey ☐ other

PREPARED WITH

☐ sugar ☐ milk ☐ cream ☐ lemon ☐ honey ☐ other

NOTES

IS THIS TEA GOOD ICED?	PURCHASED FROM	
☐ yes ☐ no		
WOULD YOU BUY AGAIN?	IDEAL FOR	RATING
☐ yes ☐ no		☆☆☆☆☆

TEA TASTING NOTES

DATE	TEA (NAME/BRAND/SELLER)	
COUNTRY OF ORIGIN:		PRICE

TEA TYPE

☐ black ☐ green ☐ white ☐ herbal ☐ oolong ☐ pu-erh ☐ fruit ☐ other

BREWING METHOD	DRY LEAVES (AMOUNT)	WATER TEMP.	STEEPING TIME(S)

TEA LEAVES	LIQUOR (COLOR)
AROMA	LIQUOR (TASTE)

AROMA CHECK LIST

☐ bitter ☐ robust ☐ nutty ☐ earthy ☐ citrus ☐ flowery ☐ sweet ☐ delicate ☐ malty

☐ spicy ☐ woodsy ☐ smokey ☐ other

PREPARED WITH

☐ sugar ☐ milk ☐ cream ☐ lemon ☐ honey ☐ other

NOTES

IS THIS TEA GOOD ICED? ☐ yes ☐ no	PURCHASED FROM	
WOULD YOU BUY AGAIN? ☐ yes ☐ no	IDEAL FOR	RATING ☆ ☆ ☆ ☆ ☆

TEA TASTING NOTES

DATE	TEA (NAME/BRAND/SELLER)		
COUNTRY OF ORIGIN:			PRICE

TEA TYPE

☐ black ☐ green ☐ white ☐ herbal ☐ oolong ☐ pu-erh ☐ fruit ☐ other

BREWING METHOD	DRY LEAVES (AMOUNT)	WATER TEMP.	STEEPING TIME(S)

TEA LEAVES	LIQUOR (COLOR)
AROMA	LIQUOR (TASTE)

AROMA CHECK LIST

☐ bitter ☐ robust ☐ nutty ☐ earthy ☐ citrus ☐ flowery ☐ sweet ☐ delicate ☐ malty

☐ spicy ☐ woodsy ☐ smokey ☐ other

PREPARED WITH

☐ sugar ☐ milk ☐ cream ☐ lemon ☐ honey ☐ other

NOTES

IS THIS TEA GOOD ICED?	PURCHASED FROM	
☐ yes ☐ no		
WOULD YOU BUY AGAIN?	IDEAL FOR	RATING
☐ yes ☐ no		☆ ☆ ☆ ☆ ☆

TEA TASTING NOTES

DATE	TEA (NAME/BRAND/SELLER)	
COUNTRY OF ORIGIN:		PRICE

TEA TYPE

☐ black ☐ green ☐ white ☐ herbal ☐ oolong ☐ pu-erh ☐ fruit ☐ other

BREWING METHOD	DRY LEAVES (AMOUNT)	WATER TEMP.	STEEPING TIME(S)

TEA LEAVES	LIQUOR (COLOR)
AROMA	LIQUOR (TASTE)

AROMA CHECK LIST

☐ bitter ☐ robust ☐ nutty ☐ earthy ☐ citrus ☐ flowery ☐ sweet ☐ delicate ☐ malty

☐ spicy ☐ woodsy ☐ smokey ☐ other

PREPARED WITH

☐ sugar ☐ milk ☐ cream ☐ lemon ☐ honey ☐ other

NOTES

IS THIS TEA GOOD ICED? ☐ yes ☐ no	PURCHASED FROM	
WOULD YOU BUY AGAIN? ☐ yes ☐ no	IDEAL FOR	RATING ☆☆☆☆☆

TEA TASTING NOTES

DATE	TEA (NAME/BRAND/SELLER)	
COUNTRY OF ORIGIN:		PRICE

TEA TYPE

☐ black ☐ green ☐ white ☐ herbal ☐ oolong ☐ pu-erh ☐ fruit ☐ other

BREWING METHOD	DRY LEAVES (AMOUNT)	WATER TEMP.	STEEPING TIME(S)

TEA LEAVES	LIQUOR (COLOR)
AROMA	LIQUOR (TASTE)

AROMA CHECK LIST

☐ bitter ☐ robust ☐ nutty ☐ earthy ☐ citrus ☐ flowery ☐ sweet ☐ delicate ☐ malty
☐ spicy ☐ woodsy ☐ smokey ☐ other

PREPARED WITH

☐ sugar ☐ milk ☐ cream ☐ lemon ☐ honey ☐ other

NOTES

IS THIS TEA GOOD ICED?	PURCHASED FROM	
☐ yes ☐ no		
WOULD YOU BUY AGAIN?	IDEAL FOR	RATING
☐ yes ☐ no		☆☆☆☆☆

TEA TASTING NOTES

DATE	TEA (NAME/BRAND/SELLER)	
COUNTRY OF ORIGIN:		PRICE

TEA TYPE

☐ black ☐ green ☐ white ☐ herbal ☐ oolong ☐ pu-erh ☐ fruit ☐ other

BREWING METHOD	DRY LEAVES (AMOUNT)	WATER TEMP.	STEEPING TIME(S)

TEA LEAVES	LIQUOR (COLOR)

AROMA	LIQUOR (TASTE)

AROMA CHECK LIST

☐ bitter ☐ robust ☐ nutty ☐ earthy ☐ citrus ☐ flowery ☐ sweet ☐ delicate ☐ malty
☐ spicy ☐ woodsy ☐ smokey ☐ other

PREPARED WITH

☐ sugar ☐ milk ☐ cream ☐ lemon ☐ honey ☐ other

NOTES

IS THIS TEA GOOD ICED? ☐ yes ☐ no	PURCHASED FROM	
WOULD YOU BUY AGAIN? ☐ yes ☐ no	IDEAL FOR	RATING ☆☆☆☆☆

TEA TASTING NOTES

DATE	TEA (NAME/BRAND/SELLER)	
COUNTRY OF ORIGIN:		PRICE

TEA TYPE

☐ black ☐ green ☐ white ☐ herbal ☐ oolong ☐ pu-erh ☐ fruit ☐ other

BREWING METHOD	DRY LEAVES (AMOUNT)	WATER TEMP.	STEEPING TIME(S)

TEA LEAVES	LIQUOR (COLOR)
AROMA	LIQUOR (TASTE)

AROMA CHECK LIST

☐ bitter ☐ robust ☐ nutty ☐ earthy ☐ citrus ☐ flowery ☐ sweet ☐ delicate ☐ malty
☐ spicy ☐ woodsy ☐ smokey ☐ other

PREPARED WITH

☐ sugar ☐ milk ☐ cream ☐ lemon ☐ honey ☐ other

NOTES

IS THIS TEA GOOD ICED?	PURCHASED FROM	
☐ yes ☐ no		
WOULD YOU BUY AGAIN?	IDEAL FOR	RATING
☐ yes ☐ no		☆☆☆☆☆

TEA TASTING NOTES

DATE	TEA (NAME/BRAND/SELLER)	
COUNTRY OF ORIGIN:		PRICE

TEA TYPE
☐ black ☐ green ☐ white ☐ herbal ☐ oolong ☐ pu-erh ☐ fruit ☐ other

BREWING METHOD	DRY LEAVES (AMOUNT)	WATER TEMP.	STEEPING TIME(S)

TEA LEAVES	LIQUOR (COLOR)
AROMA	LIQUOR (TASTE)

AROMA CHECK LIST
☐ bitter ☐ robust ☐ nutty ☐ earthy ☐ citrus ☐ flowery ☐ sweet ☐ delicate ☐ malty
☐ spicy ☐ woodsy ☐ smokey ☐ other

PREPARED WITH
☐ sugar ☐ milk ☐ cream ☐ lemon ☐ honey ☐ other

NOTES

IS THIS TEA GOOD ICED?	PURCHASED FROM
☐ yes ☐ no	
WOULD YOU BUY AGAIN?	IDEAL FOR	RATING
☐ yes ☐ no		☆ ☆ ☆ ☆ ☆

TEA TASTING NOTES

DATE	TEA (NAME/BRAND/SELLER)	
COUNTRY OF ORIGIN:		PRICE

TEA TYPE

☐ black ☐ green ☐ white ☐ herbal ☐ oolong ☐ pu-erh ☐ fruit ☐ other

BREWING METHOD	DRY LEAVES (AMOUNT)	WATER TEMP.	STEEPING TIME(S)

TEA LEAVES	LIQUOR (COLOR)
AROMA	LIQUOR (TASTE)

AROMA CHECK LIST

☐ bitter ☐ robust ☐ nutty ☐ earthy ☐ citrus ☐ flowery ☐ sweet ☐ delicate ☐ malty
☐ spicy ☐ woodsy ☐ smokey ☐ other

PREPARED WITH

☐ sugar ☐ milk ☐ cream ☐ lemon ☐ honey ☐ other

NOTES

IS THIS TEA GOOD ICED?	PURCHASED FROM	
☐ yes ☐ no		
WOULD YOU BUY AGAIN?	IDEAL FOR	RATING
☐ yes ☐ no		☆☆☆☆☆

TEA TASTING NOTES

DATE	TEA (NAME/BRAND/SELLER)	
COUNTRY OF ORIGIN:		PRICE

TEA TYPE
☐ black ☐ green ☐ white ☐ herbal ☐ oolong ☐ pu-erh ☐ fruit ☐ other

BREWING METHOD	DRY LEAVES (AMOUNT)	WATER TEMP.	STEEPING TIME(S)

TEA LEAVES	LIQUOR (COLOR)
AROMA	LIQUOR (TASTE)

AROMA CHECK LIST
☐ bitter ☐ robust ☐ nutty ☐ earthy ☐ citrus ☐ flowery ☐ sweet ☐ delicate ☐ malty
☐ spicy ☐ woodsy ☐ smokey ☐ other

PREPARED WITH
☐ sugar ☐ milk ☐ cream ☐ lemon ☐ honey ☐ other

NOTES

IS THIS TEA GOOD ICED? ☐ yes ☐ no	PURCHASED FROM	
WOULD YOU BUY AGAIN? ☐ yes ☐ no	IDEAL FOR	RATING ☆☆☆☆☆

TEA TASTING NOTES

DATE	TEA (NAME/BRAND/SELLER)	
COUNTRY OF ORIGIN:		PRICE

TEA TYPE

☐ black ☐ green ☐ white ☐ herbal ☐ oolong ☐ pu-erh ☐ fruit ☐ other

BREWING METHOD	DRY LEAVES (AMOUNT)	WATER TEMP.	STEEPING TIME(S)

TEA LEAVES	LIQUOR (COLOR)
AROMA	LIQUOR (TASTE)

AROMA CHECK LIST

☐ bitter ☐ robust ☐ nutty ☐ earthy ☐ citrus ☐ flowery ☐ sweet ☐ delicate ☐ malty
☐ spicy ☐ woodsy ☐ smokey ☐ other

PREPARED WITH

☐ sugar ☐ milk ☐ cream ☐ lemon ☐ honey ☐ other

NOTES

IS THIS TEA GOOD ICED?	PURCHASED FROM	
☐ yes ☐ no		
WOULD YOU BUY AGAIN?	IDEAL FOR	RATING
☐ yes ☐ no		☆☆☆☆☆

TEA TASTING NOTES

DATE	TEA (NAME/BRAND/SELLER)	
COUNTRY OF ORIGIN:		PRICE

TEA TYPE
☐ black ☐ green ☐ white ☐ herbal ☐ oolong ☐ pu-erh ☐ fruit ☐ other

BREWING METHOD	DRY LEAVES (AMOUNT)	WATER TEMP.	STEEPING TIME(S)

TEA LEAVES	LIQUOR (COLOR)
AROMA	LIQUOR (TASTE)

AROMA CHECK LIST
☐ bitter ☐ robust ☐ nutty ☐ earthy ☐ citrus ☐ flowery ☐ sweet ☐ delicate ☐ malty
☐ spicy ☐ woodsy ☐ smokey ☐ other

PREPARED WITH
☐ sugar ☐ milk ☐ cream ☐ lemon ☐ honey ☐ other

NOTES

IS THIS TEA GOOD ICED?	PURCHASED FROM	
☐ yes ☐ no		
WOULD YOU BUY AGAIN?	IDEAL FOR	RATING
☐ yes ☐ no		☆ ☆ ☆ ☆ ☆

TEA TASTING NOTES

DATE	TEA (NAME/BRAND/SELLER)	
COUNTRY OF ORIGIN:		PRICE

TEA TYPE

☐ black   ☐ green   ☐ white   ☐ herbal   ☐ oolong   ☐ pu-erh   ☐ fruit   ☐ other

BREWING METHOD	DRY LEAVES (AMOUNT)	WATER TEMP.	STEEPING TIME(S)

TEA LEAVES	LIQUOR (COLOR)
AROMA	LIQUOR (TASTE)

AROMA CHECK LIST

☐ bitter   ☐ robust   ☐ nutty   ☐ earthy   ☐ citrus   ☐ flowery   ☐ sweet   ☐ delicate   ☐ malty
☐ spicy   ☐ woodsy   ☐ smokey   ☐ other

PREPARED WITH

☐ sugar   ☐ milk   ☐ cream   ☐ lemon   ☐ honey   ☐ other

NOTES

IS THIS TEA GOOD ICED? ☐ yes ☐ no	PURCHASED FROM	
WOULD YOU BUY AGAIN? ☐ yes ☐ no	IDEAL FOR	RATING ☆☆☆☆☆

TEA TASTING NOTES

DATE	TEA (NAME/BRAND/SELLER)	
COUNTRY OF ORIGIN:		PRICE

TEA TYPE

☐ black   ☐ green   ☐ white   ☐ herbal   ☐ oolong   ☐ pu-erh   ☐ fruit   ☐ other

BREWING METHOD	DRY LEAVES (AMOUNT)	WATER TEMP.	STEEPING TIME(S)

TEA LEAVES	LIQUOR (COLOR)
AROMA	LIQUOR (TASTE)

AROMA CHECK LIST

☐ bitter   ☐ robust   ☐ nutty   ☐ earthy   ☐ citrus   ☐ flowery   ☐ sweet   ☐ delicate   ☐ malty
☐ spicy   ☐ woodsy   ☐ smokey   ☐ other

PREPARED WITH

☐ sugar   ☐ milk   ☐ cream   ☐ lemon   ☐ honey   ☐ other

NOTES

IS THIS TEA GOOD ICED? ☐ yes ☐ no	PURCHASED FROM	
WOULD YOU BUY AGAIN? ☐ yes ☐ no	IDEAL FOR	RATING ☆☆☆☆☆

TEA TASTING NOTES

DATE	TEA (NAME/BRAND/SELLER)	
COUNTRY OF ORIGIN:		PRICE

TEA TYPE
☐ black ☐ green ☐ white ☐ herbal ☐ oolong ☐ pu-erh ☐ fruit ☐ other

BREWING METHOD	DRY LEAVES (AMOUNT)	WATER TEMP.	STEEPING TIME(S)

TEA LEAVES	LIQUOR (COLOR)
AROMA	LIQUOR (TASTE)

AROMA CHECK LIST
☐ bitter ☐ robust ☐ nutty ☐ earthy ☐ citrus ☐ flowery ☐ sweet ☐ delicate ☐ malty
☐ spicy ☐ woodsy ☐ smokey ☐ other

PREPARED WITH
☐ sugar ☐ milk ☐ cream ☐ lemon ☐ honey ☐ other

NOTES

IS THIS TEA GOOD ICED?	PURCHASED FROM	
☐ yes ☐ no		
WOULD YOU BUY AGAIN?	IDEAL FOR	RATING
☐ yes ☐ no		☆ ☆ ☆ ☆ ☆

TEA TASTING NOTES

DATE	TEA (NAME/BRAND/SELLER)	
COUNTRY OF ORIGIN:		PRICE

TEA TYPE
☐ black ☐ green ☐ white ☐ herbal ☐ oolong ☐ pu-erh ☐ fruit ☐ other

BREWING METHOD	DRY LEAVES (AMOUNT)	WATER TEMP.	STEEPING TIME(S)

TEA LEAVES	LIQUOR (COLOR)
AROMA	LIQUOR (TASTE)

AROMA CHECK LIST
☐ bitter ☐ robust ☐ nutty ☐ earthy ☐ citrus ☐ flowery ☐ sweet ☐ delicate ☐ malty
☐ spicy ☐ woodsy ☐ smokey ☐ other

PREPARED WITH
☐ sugar ☐ milk ☐ cream ☐ lemon ☐ honey ☐ other

NOTES

IS THIS TEA GOOD ICED?	PURCHASED FROM	
☐ yes ☐ no		
WOULD YOU BUY AGAIN?	IDEAL FOR	RATING
☐ yes ☐ no		☆ ☆ ☆ ☆ ☆

TEA TASTING NOTES

DATE	TEA (NAME/BRAND/SELLER)		
COUNTRY OF ORIGIN:			PRICE

TEA TYPE

☐ black   ☐ green   ☐ white   ☐ herbal   ☐ oolong   ☐ pu-erh   ☐ fruit   ☐ other

BREWING METHOD	DRY LEAVES (AMOUNT)	WATER TEMP.	STEEPING TIME(S)

TEA LEAVES	LIQUOR (COLOR)
AROMA	LIQUOR (TASTE)

AROMA CHECK LIST

☐ bitter   ☐ robust   ☐ nutty   ☐ earthy   ☐ citrus   ☐ flowery   ☐ sweet   ☐ delicate   ☐ malty
☐ spicy   ☐ woodsy   ☐ smokey   ☐ other

PREPARED WITH

☐ sugar   ☐ milk   ☐ cream   ☐ lemon   ☐ honey   ☐ other

NOTES

IS THIS TEA GOOD ICED? ☐ yes ☐ no	PURCHASED FROM	
WOULD YOU BUY AGAIN? ☐ yes ☐ no	IDEAL FOR	RATING ☆☆☆☆☆

TEA TASTING NOTES

DATE	TEA (NAME/BRAND/SELLER)	
COUNTRY OF ORIGIN:		PRICE

TEA TYPE

☐ black ☐ green ☐ white ☐ herbal ☐ oolong ☐ pu-erh ☐ fruit ☐ other

BREWING METHOD	DRY LEAVES (AMOUNT)	WATER TEMP.	STEEPING TIME(S)

TEA LEAVES	LIQUOR (COLOR)
AROMA	LIQUOR (TASTE)

AROMA CHECK LIST

☐ bitter ☐ robust ☐ nutty ☐ earthy ☐ citrus ☐ flowery ☐ sweet ☐ delicate ☐ malty
☐ spicy ☐ woodsy ☐ smokey ☐ other

PREPARED WITH

☐ sugar ☐ milk ☐ cream ☐ lemon ☐ honey ☐ other

NOTES

IS THIS TEA GOOD ICED?	PURCHASED FROM	
☐ yes ☐ no		
WOULD YOU BUY AGAIN?	IDEAL FOR	RATING
☐ yes ☐ no		☆☆☆☆☆

TEA TASTING NOTES

DATE	TEA (NAME/BRAND/SELLER)	
COUNTRY OF ORIGIN:		PRICE

TEA TYPE

☐ black ☐ green ☐ white ☐ herbal ☐ oolong ☐ pu-erh ☐ fruit ☐ other

BREWING METHOD	DRY LEAVES (AMOUNT)	WATER TEMP.	STEEPING TIME(S)

TEA LEAVES	LIQUOR (COLOR)
AROMA	LIQUOR (TASTE)

AROMA CHECK LIST

☐ bitter ☐ robust ☐ nutty ☐ earthy ☐ citrus ☐ flowery ☐ sweet ☐ delicate ☐ malty
☐ spicy ☐ woodsy ☐ smokey ☐ other

PREPARED WITH

☐ sugar ☐ milk ☐ cream ☐ lemon ☐ honey ☐ other

NOTES

IS THIS TEA GOOD ICED?	PURCHASED FROM	
☐ yes ☐ no		
WOULD YOU BUY AGAIN?	IDEAL FOR	RATING
☐ yes ☐ no		☆☆☆☆☆

TEA TASTING NOTES

DATE	TEA (NAME/BRAND/SELLER)	
COUNTRY OF ORIGIN:		PRICE

TEA TYPE

☐ black ☐ green ☐ white ☐ herbal ☐ oolong ☐ pu-erh ☐ fruit ☐ other

BREWING METHOD	DRY LEAVES (AMOUNT)	WATER TEMP.	STEEPING TIME(S)

TEA LEAVES	LIQUOR (COLOR)
AROMA	LIQUOR (TASTE)

AROMA CHECK LIST

☐ bitter ☐ robust ☐ nutty ☐ earthy ☐ citrus ☐ flowery ☐ sweet ☐ delicate ☐ malty
☐ spicy ☐ woodsy ☐ smokey ☐ other

PREPARED WITH

☐ sugar ☐ milk ☐ cream ☐ lemon ☐ honey ☐ other

NOTES

IS THIS TEA GOOD ICED? ☐ yes ☐ no	PURCHASED FROM	
WOULD YOU BUY AGAIN? ☐ yes ☐ no	IDEAL FOR	RATING ☆ ☆ ☆ ☆ ☆

TEA TASTING NOTES

DATE	TEA (NAME/BRAND/SELLER)		
COUNTRY OF ORIGIN:			PRICE

TEA TYPE

☐ black ☐ green ☐ white ☐ herbal ☐ oolong ☐ pu-erh ☐ fruit ☐ other

BREWING METHOD	DRY LEAVES (AMOUNT)	WATER TEMP.	STEEPING TIME(S)

TEA LEAVES	LIQUOR (COLOR)
AROMA	LIQUOR (TASTE)

AROMA CHECK LIST

☐ bitter ☐ robust ☐ nutty ☐ earthy ☐ citrus ☐ flowery ☐ sweet ☐ delicate ☐ malty
☐ spicy ☐ woodsy ☐ smokey ☐ other

PREPARED WITH

☐ sugar ☐ milk ☐ cream ☐ lemon ☐ honey ☐ other

NOTES

IS THIS TEA GOOD ICED?	PURCHASED FROM		
☐ yes ☐ no			
WOULD YOU BUY AGAIN?	IDEAL FOR		RATING
☐ yes ☐ no			☆☆☆☆☆

TEA TASTING NOTES

DATE	TEA (NAME/BRAND/SELLER)	
COUNTRY OF ORIGIN:		PRICE

TEA TYPE

☐ black ☐ green ☐ white ☐ herbal ☐ oolong ☐ pu-erh ☐ fruit ☐ other

BREWING METHOD	DRY LEAVES (AMOUNT)	WATER TEMP.	STEEPING TIME(S)

TEA LEAVES	LIQUOR (COLOR)
AROMA	LIQUOR (TASTE)

AROMA CHECK LIST

☐ bitter ☐ robust ☐ nutty ☐ earthy ☐ citrus ☐ flowery ☐ sweet ☐ delicate ☐ malty
☐ spicy ☐ woodsy ☐ smokey ☐ other

PREPARED WITH

☐ sugar ☐ milk ☐ cream ☐ lemon ☐ honey ☐ other

NOTES

IS THIS TEA GOOD ICED? ☐ yes ☐ no	PURCHASED FROM	
WOULD YOU BUY AGAIN? ☐ yes ☐ no	IDEAL FOR	RATING ☆☆☆☆☆

TEA TASTING NOTES

DATE	TEA (NAME/BRAND/SELLER)	
COUNTRY OF ORIGIN:		PRICE

TEA TYPE

☐ black ☐ green ☐ white ☐ herbal ☐ oolong ☐ pu-erh ☐ fruit ☐ other

BREWING METHOD	DRY LEAVES (AMOUNT)	WATER TEMP.	STEEPING TIME(S)

TEA LEAVES	LIQUOR (COLOR)
AROMA	LIQUOR (TASTE)

AROMA CHECK LIST

☐ bitter ☐ robust ☐ nutty ☐ earthy ☐ citrus ☐ flowery ☐ sweet ☐ delicate ☐ malty
☐ spicy ☐ woodsy ☐ smokey ☐ other

PREPARED WITH

☐ sugar ☐ milk ☐ cream ☐ lemon ☐ honey ☐ other

NOTES

IS THIS TEA GOOD ICED?	PURCHASED FROM	
☐ yes ☐ no		
WOULD YOU BUY AGAIN?	IDEAL FOR	RATING
☐ yes ☐ no		☆ ☆ ☆ ☆ ☆

TEA TASTING NOTES

DATE	TEA (NAME/BRAND/SELLER)		
COUNTRY OF ORIGIN:			PRICE

TEA TYPE

☐ black ☐ green ☐ white ☐ herbal ☐ oolong ☐ pu-erh ☐ fruit ☐ other

BREWING METHOD	DRY LEAVES (AMOUNT)	WATER TEMP.	STEEPING TIME(S)

TEA LEAVES	LIQUOR (COLOR)
AROMA	LIQUOR (TASTE)

AROMA CHECK LIST

☐ bitter ☐ robust ☐ nutty ☐ earthy ☐ citrus ☐ flowery ☐ sweet ☐ delicate ☐ malty
☐ spicy ☐ woodsy ☐ smokey ☐ other

PREPARED WITH

☐ sugar ☐ milk ☐ cream ☐ lemon ☐ honey ☐ other

NOTES

IS THIS TEA GOOD ICED?	PURCHASED FROM	
☐ yes ☐ no		
WOULD YOU BUY AGAIN?	IDEAL FOR	RATING
☐ yes ☐ no		☆☆☆☆☆

TEA TASTING NOTES

DATE	TEA (NAME/BRAND/SELLER)		
COUNTRY OF ORIGIN:			PRICE

TEA TYPE

☐ black ☐ green ☐ white ☐ herbal ☐ oolong ☐ pu-erh ☐ fruit ☐ other

BREWING METHOD	DRY LEAVES (AMOUNT)	WATER TEMP.	STEEPING TIME(S)

TEA LEAVES	LIQUOR (COLOR)
AROMA	LIQUOR (TASTE)

AROMA CHECK LIST

☐ bitter ☐ robust ☐ nutty ☐ earthy ☐ citrus ☐ flowery ☐ sweet ☐ delicate ☐ malty
☐ spicy ☐ woodsy ☐ smokey ☐ other

PREPARED WITH

☐ sugar ☐ milk ☐ cream ☐ lemon ☐ honey ☐ other

NOTES

IS THIS TEA GOOD ICED?	PURCHASED FROM	
☐ yes ☐ no		
WOULD YOU BUY AGAIN?	IDEAL FOR	RATING
☐ yes ☐ no		☆ ☆ ☆ ☆ ☆

TEA TASTING NOTES

DATE	TEA (NAME/BRAND/SELLER)	
COUNTRY OF ORIGIN:		PRICE

TEA TYPE

☐ black   ☐ green   ☐ white   ☐ herbal   ☐ oolong   ☐ pu-erh   ☐ fruit   ☐ other

BREWING METHOD	DRY LEAVES (AMOUNT)	WATER TEMP.	STEEPING TIME(S)

TEA LEAVES	LIQUOR (COLOR)
AROMA	LIQUOR (TASTE)

AROMA CHECK LIST

☐ bitter   ☐ robust   ☐ nutty   ☐ earthy   ☐ citrus   ☐ flowery   ☐ sweet   ☐ delicate   ☐ malty
☐ spicy   ☐ woodsy   ☐ smokey   ☐ other

PREPARED WITH

☐ sugar   ☐ milk   ☐ cream   ☐ lemon   ☐ honey   ☐ other

NOTES

IS THIS TEA GOOD ICED? ☐ yes ☐ no	PURCHASED FROM	
WOULD YOU BUY AGAIN? ☐ yes ☐ no	IDEAL FOR	RATING ☆ ☆ ☆ ☆ ☆

TEA TASTING NOTES

DATE	TEA (NAME/BRAND/SELLER)	
COUNTRY OF ORIGIN:		PRICE

TEA TYPE

☐ black ☐ green ☐ white ☐ herbal ☐ oolong ☐ pu-erh ☐ fruit ☐ other

BREWING METHOD	DRY LEAVES (AMOUNT)	WATER TEMP.	STEEPING TIME(S)

TEA LEAVES	LIQUOR (COLOR)
AROMA	LIQUOR (TASTE)

AROMA CHECK LIST

☐ bitter ☐ robust ☐ nutty ☐ earthy ☐ citrus ☐ flowery ☐ sweet ☐ delicate ☐ malty
☐ spicy ☐ woodsy ☐ smokey ☐ other

PREPARED WITH

☐ sugar ☐ milk ☐ cream ☐ lemon ☐ honey ☐ other

NOTES

IS THIS TEA GOOD ICED?	PURCHASED FROM	
☐ yes ☐ no		
WOULD YOU BUY AGAIN?	IDEAL FOR	RATING
☐ yes ☐ no		☆☆☆☆☆

TEA TASTING NOTES

DATE	TEA (NAME/BRAND/SELLER)		
COUNTRY OF ORIGIN:			PRICE
TEA TYPE ☐ black ☐ green ☐ white ☐ herbal ☐ oolong ☐ pu-erh ☐ fruit ☐ other			
BREWING METHOD	DRY LEAVES (AMOUNT)	WATER TEMP.	STEEPING TIME(S)
TEA LEAVES		LIQUOR (COLOR)	
AROMA		LIQUOR (TASTE)	
AROMA CHECK LIST ☐ bitter ☐ robust ☐ nutty ☐ earthy ☐ citrus ☐ flowery ☐ sweet ☐ delicate ☐ malty ☐ spicy ☐ woodsy ☐ smokey ☐ other			
PREPARED WITH ☐ sugar ☐ milk ☐ cream ☐ lemon ☐ honey ☐ other			
NOTES			
IS THIS TEA GOOD ICED? ☐ yes ☐ no	PURCHASED FROM		
WOULD YOU BUY AGAIN? ☐ yes ☐ no	IDEAL FOR	RATING ☆☆☆☆☆	

TEA TASTING NOTES

DATE	TEA (NAME/BRAND/SELLER)	
COUNTRY OF ORIGIN:		PRICE

TEA TYPE

☐ black   ☐ green   ☐ white   ☐ herbal   ☐ oolong   ☐ pu-erh   ☐ fruit   ☐ other

BREWING METHOD	DRY LEAVES (AMOUNT)	WATER TEMP.	STEEPING TIME(S)

TEA LEAVES	LIQUOR (COLOR)

AROMA	LIQUOR (TASTE)

AROMA CHECK LIST

☐ bitter   ☐ robust   ☐ nutty   ☐ earthy   ☐ citrus   ☐ flowery   ☐ sweet   ☐ delicate   ☐ malty
☐ spicy   ☐ woodsy   ☐ smokey   ☐ other

PREPARED WITH

☐ sugar   ☐ milk   ☐ cream   ☐ lemon   ☐ honey   ☐ other

NOTES

IS THIS TEA GOOD ICED?	PURCHASED FROM	
☐ yes ☐ no		
WOULD YOU BUY AGAIN?	IDEAL FOR	RATING
☐ yes ☐ no		☆☆☆☆☆

TEA TASTING NOTES

DATE	TEA (NAME/BRAND/SELLER)	
COUNTRY OF ORIGIN:		PRICE

TEA TYPE

☐ black ☐ green ☐ white ☐ herbal ☐ oolong ☐ pu-erh ☐ fruit ☐ other

BREWING METHOD	DRY LEAVES (AMOUNT)	WATER TEMP.	STEEPING TIME(S)

TEA LEAVES	LIQUOR (COLOR)
AROMA	LIQUOR (TASTE)

AROMA CHECK LIST

☐ bitter ☐ robust ☐ nutty ☐ earthy ☐ citrus ☐ flowery ☐ sweet ☐ delicate ☐ malty
☐ spicy ☐ woodsy ☐ smokey ☐ other

PREPARED WITH

☐ sugar ☐ milk ☐ cream ☐ lemon ☐ honey ☐ other

NOTES

IS THIS TEA GOOD ICED?	PURCHASED FROM	
☐ yes ☐ no		
WOULD YOU BUY AGAIN?	IDEAL FOR	RATING
☐ yes ☐ no		☆ ☆ ☆ ☆ ☆

TEA TASTING NOTES

DATE	TEA (NAME/BRAND/SELLER)	
COUNTRY OF ORIGIN:		PRICE

TEA TYPE

☐ black ☐ green ☐ white ☐ herbal ☐ oolong ☐ pu-erh ☐ fruit ☐ other

BREWING METHOD	DRY LEAVES (AMOUNT)	WATER TEMP.	STEEPING TIME(S)

TEA LEAVES	LIQUOR (COLOR)
AROMA	LIQUOR (TASTE)

AROMA CHECK LIST

☐ bitter ☐ robust ☐ nutty ☐ earthy ☐ citrus ☐ flowery ☐ sweet ☐ delicate ☐ malty
☐ spicy ☐ woodsy ☐ smokey ☐ other

PREPARED WITH

☐ sugar ☐ milk ☐ cream ☐ lemon ☐ honey ☐ other

NOTES

IS THIS TEA GOOD ICED? ☐ yes ☐ no	PURCHASED FROM	
WOULD YOU BUY AGAIN? ☐ yes ☐ no	IDEAL FOR	RATING ☆ ☆ ☆ ☆ ☆

TEA TASTING NOTES

DATE	TEA (NAME/BRAND/SELLER)	
COUNTRY OF ORIGIN:		PRICE

TEA TYPE

☐ black ☐ green ☐ white ☐ herbal ☐ oolong ☐ pu-erh ☐ fruit ☐ other

BREWING METHOD	DRY LEAVES (AMOUNT)	WATER TEMP.	STEEPING TIME(S)

TEA LEAVES	LIQUOR (COLOR)
AROMA	LIQUOR (TASTE)

AROMA CHECK LIST

☐ bitter ☐ robust ☐ nutty ☐ earthy ☐ citrus ☐ flowery ☐ sweet ☐ delicate ☐ malty

☐ spicy ☐ woodsy ☐ smokey ☐ other

PREPARED WITH

☐ sugar ☐ milk ☐ cream ☐ lemon ☐ honey ☐ other

NOTES

IS THIS TEA GOOD ICED?	PURCHASED FROM	
☐ yes ☐ no		
WOULD YOU BUY AGAIN?	IDEAL FOR	RATING
☐ yes ☐ no		☆ ☆ ☆ ☆ ☆

TEA TASTING NOTES

DATE	TEA (NAME/BRAND/SELLER)	
COUNTRY OF ORIGIN:		PRICE

TEA TYPE

☐ black   ☐ green   ☐ white   ☐ herbal   ☐ oolong   ☐ pu-erh   ☐ fruit   ☐ other

BREWING METHOD	DRY LEAVES (AMOUNT)	WATER TEMP.	STEEPING TIME(S)

TEA LEAVES	LIQUOR (COLOR)
AROMA	LIQUOR (TASTE)

AROMA CHECK LIST

☐ bitter   ☐ robust   ☐ nutty   ☐ earthy   ☐ citrus   ☐ flowery   ☐ sweet   ☐ delicate   ☐ malty
☐ spicy   ☐ woodsy   ☐ smokey   ☐ other

PREPARED WITH

☐ sugar   ☐ milk   ☐ cream   ☐ lemon   ☐ honey   ☐ other

NOTES

IS THIS TEA GOOD ICED?	PURCHASED FROM	
☐ yes ☐ no		
WOULD YOU BUY AGAIN?	IDEAL FOR	RATING
☐ yes ☐ no		☆☆☆☆☆

TEA TASTING NOTES

DATE	TEA (NAME/BRAND/SELLER)	
COUNTRY OF ORIGIN:		PRICE

TEA TYPE

☐ black ☐ green ☐ white ☐ herbal ☐ oolong ☐ pu-erh ☐ fruit ☐ other

BREWING METHOD	DRY LEAVES (AMOUNT)	WATER TEMP.	STEEPING TIME(S)

TEA LEAVES	LIQUOR (COLOR)
AROMA	LIQUOR (TASTE)

AROMA CHECK LIST

☐ bitter ☐ robust ☐ nutty ☐ earthy ☐ citrus ☐ flowery ☐ sweet ☐ delicate ☐ malty

☐ spicy ☐ woodsy ☐ smokey ☐ other

PREPARED WITH

☐ sugar ☐ milk ☐ cream ☐ lemon ☐ honey ☐ other

NOTES

IS THIS TEA GOOD ICED?	PURCHASED FROM	
☐ yes ☐ no		
WOULD YOU BUY AGAIN?	IDEAL FOR	RATING
☐ yes ☐ no		☆☆☆☆☆

TEA TASTING NOTES

DATE	TEA (NAME/BRAND/SELLER)		
COUNTRY OF ORIGIN:			PRICE

TEA TYPE

☐ black ☐ green ☐ white ☐ herbal ☐ oolong ☐ pu-erh ☐ fruit ☐ other

BREWING METHOD	DRY LEAVES (AMOUNT)	WATER TEMP.	STEEPING TIME(S)

TEA LEAVES	LIQUOR (COLOR)

AROMA	LIQUOR (TASTE)

AROMA CHECK LIST

☐ bitter ☐ robust ☐ nutty ☐ earthy ☐ citrus ☐ flowery ☐ sweet ☐ delicate ☐ malty
☐ spicy ☐ woodsy ☐ smokey ☐ other

PREPARED WITH

☐ sugar ☐ milk ☐ cream ☐ lemon ☐ honey ☐ other

NOTES

IS THIS TEA GOOD ICED? ☐ yes ☐ no	PURCHASED FROM		
WOULD YOU BUY AGAIN? ☐ yes ☐ no	IDEAL FOR		RATING ☆☆☆☆☆

TEA TASTING NOTES

DATE	TEA (NAME/BRAND/SELLER)	
COUNTRY OF ORIGIN:		PRICE

TEA TYPE

☐ black ☐ green ☐ white ☐ herbal ☐ oolong ☐ pu-erh ☐ fruit ☐ other

BREWING METHOD	DRY LEAVES (AMOUNT)	WATER TEMP.	STEEPING TIME(S)

TEA LEAVES	LIQUOR (COLOR)
AROMA	LIQUOR (TASTE)

AROMA CHECK LIST

☐ bitter ☐ robust ☐ nutty ☐ earthy ☐ citrus ☐ flowery ☐ sweet ☐ delicate ☐ malty
☐ spicy ☐ woodsy ☐ smokey ☐ other

PREPARED WITH

☐ sugar ☐ milk ☐ cream ☐ lemon ☐ honey ☐ other

NOTES

IS THIS TEA GOOD ICED?	PURCHASED FROM
☐ yes ☐ no	

WOULD YOU BUY AGAIN?	IDEAL FOR	RATING
☐ yes ☐ no		☆ ☆ ☆ ☆ ☆

TEA TASTING NOTES

DATE	TEA (NAME/BRAND/SELLER)	
COUNTRY OF ORIGIN:		PRICE

TEA TYPE

☐ black   ☐ green   ☐ white   ☐ herbal   ☐ oolong   ☐ pu-erh   ☐ fruit   ☐ other

BREWING METHOD	DRY LEAVES (AMOUNT)	WATER TEMP.	STEEPING TIME(S)

TEA LEAVES	LIQUOR (COLOR)
AROMA	LIQUOR (TASTE)

AROMA CHECK LIST

☐ bitter   ☐ robust   ☐ nutty   ☐ earthy   ☐ citrus   ☐ flowery   ☐ sweet   ☐ delicate   ☐ malty
☐ spicy   ☐ woodsy   ☐ smokey   ☐ other

PREPARED WITH

☐ sugar   ☐ milk   ☐ cream   ☐ lemon   ☐ honey   ☐ other

NOTES

IS THIS TEA GOOD ICED? ☐ yes ☐ no	PURCHASED FROM	
WOULD YOU BUY AGAIN? ☐ yes ☐ no	IDEAL FOR	RATING ☆☆☆☆☆

TEA TASTING NOTES

DATE	TEA (NAME/BRAND/SELLER)	
COUNTRY OF ORIGIN:		PRICE

TEA TYPE

☐ black ☐ green ☐ white ☐ herbal ☐ oolong ☐ pu-erh ☐ fruit ☐ other

BREWING METHOD	DRY LEAVES (AMOUNT)	WATER TEMP.	STEEPING TIME(S)

TEA LEAVES	LIQUOR (COLOR)
AROMA	LIQUOR (TASTE)

AROMA CHECK LIST

☐ bitter ☐ robust ☐ nutty ☐ earthy ☐ citrus ☐ flowery ☐ sweet ☐ delicate ☐ malty
☐ spicy ☐ woodsy ☐ smokey ☐ other

PREPARED WITH

☐ sugar ☐ milk ☐ cream ☐ lemon ☐ honey ☐ other

NOTES

IS THIS TEA GOOD ICED?	PURCHASED FROM	
☐ yes ☐ no		
WOULD YOU BUY AGAIN?	IDEAL FOR	RATING
☐ yes ☐ no		☆☆☆☆☆

TEA TASTING NOTES

DATE	TEA (NAME/BRAND/SELLER)		
COUNTRY OF ORIGIN:			PRICE
TEA TYPE ☐ black ☐ green ☐ white ☐ herbal ☐ oolong ☐ pu-erh ☐ fruit ☐ other			
BREWING METHOD	DRY LEAVES (AMOUNT)	WATER TEMP.	STEEPING TIME(S)

TEA LEAVES	LIQUOR (COLOR)
AROMA	LIQUOR (TASTE)

AROMA CHECK LIST
☐ bitter ☐ robust ☐ nutty ☐ earthy ☐ citrus ☐ flowery ☐ sweet ☐ delicate ☐ malty
☐ spicy ☐ woodsy ☐ smokey ☐ other

PREPARED WITH
☐ sugar ☐ milk ☐ cream ☐ lemon ☐ honey ☐ other

NOTES

IS THIS TEA GOOD ICED? ☐ yes ☐ no	PURCHASED FROM	
WOULD YOU BUY AGAIN? ☐ yes ☐ no	IDEAL FOR	RATING ☆☆☆☆☆

TEA TASTING NOTES

DATE	TEA (NAME/BRAND/SELLER)	
COUNTRY OF ORIGIN:		PRICE

TEA TYPE

☐ black ☐ green ☐ white ☐ herbal ☐ oolong ☐ pu-erh ☐ fruit ☐ other

BREWING METHOD	DRY LEAVES (AMOUNT)	WATER TEMP.	STEEPING TIME(S)

TEA LEAVES	LIQUOR (COLOR)
AROMA	LIQUOR (TASTE)

AROMA CHECK LIST

☐ bitter ☐ robust ☐ nutty ☐ earthy ☐ citrus ☐ flowery ☐ sweet ☐ delicate ☐ malty
☐ spicy ☐ woodsy ☐ smokey ☐ other

PREPARED WITH

☐ sugar ☐ milk ☐ cream ☐ lemon ☐ honey ☐ other

NOTES

IS THIS TEA GOOD ICED? ☐ yes ☐ no	PURCHASED FROM	
WOULD YOU BUY AGAIN? ☐ yes ☐ no	IDEAL FOR	RATING ☆☆☆☆☆

TEA TASTING NOTES

DATE	TEA (NAME/BRAND/SELLER)	
COUNTRY OF ORIGIN:		PRICE

TEA TYPE

☐ black ☐ green ☐ white ☐ herbal ☐ oolong ☐ pu-erh ☐ fruit ☐ other

BREWING METHOD	DRY LEAVES (AMOUNT)	WATER TEMP.	STEEPING TIME(S)

TEA LEAVES	LIQUOR (COLOR)
AROMA	LIQUOR (TASTE)

AROMA CHECK LIST

☐ bitter ☐ robust ☐ nutty ☐ earthy ☐ citrus ☐ flowery ☐ sweet ☐ delicate ☐ malty

☐ spicy ☐ woodsy ☐ smokey ☐ other

PREPARED WITH

☐ sugar ☐ milk ☐ cream ☐ lemon ☐ honey ☐ other

NOTES

IS THIS TEA GOOD ICED?	PURCHASED FROM	
☐ yes ☐ no		
WOULD YOU BUY AGAIN?	IDEAL FOR	RATING
☐ yes ☐ no		☆ ☆ ☆ ☆ ☆

TEA TASTING NOTES

DATE	TEA (NAME/BRAND/SELLER)	
COUNTRY OF ORIGIN:		PRICE

TEA TYPE

☐ black ☐ green ☐ white ☐ herbal ☐ oolong ☐ pu-erh ☐ fruit ☐ other

BREWING METHOD	DRY LEAVES (AMOUNT)	WATER TEMP.	STEEPING TIME(S)

TEA LEAVES	LIQUOR (COLOR)
AROMA	LIQUOR (TASTE)

AROMA CHECK LIST

☐ bitter ☐ robust ☐ nutty ☐ earthy ☐ citrus ☐ flowery ☐ sweet ☐ delicate ☐ malty

☐ spicy ☐ woodsy ☐ smokey ☐ other

PREPARED WITH

☐ sugar ☐ milk ☐ cream ☐ lemon ☐ honey ☐ other

NOTES

IS THIS TEA GOOD ICED?	PURCHASED FROM	
☐ yes ☐ no		
WOULD YOU BUY AGAIN?	IDEAL FOR	RATING
☐ yes ☐ no		☆☆☆☆☆

TEA TASTING NOTES

DATE	TEA (NAME/BRAND/SELLER)		
COUNTRY OF ORIGIN:			PRICE

TEA TYPE

☐ black ☐ green ☐ white ☐ herbal ☐ oolong ☐ pu-erh ☐ fruit ☐ other

BREWING METHOD	DRY LEAVES (AMOUNT)	WATER TEMP.	STEEPING TIME(S)

TEA LEAVES	LIQUOR (COLOR)
AROMA	LIQUOR (TASTE)

AROMA CHECK LIST

☐ bitter ☐ robust ☐ nutty ☐ earthy ☐ citrus ☐ flowery ☐ sweet ☐ delicate ☐ malty
☐ spicy ☐ woodsy ☐ smokey ☐ other

PREPARED WITH

☐ sugar ☐ milk ☐ cream ☐ lemon ☐ honey ☐ other

NOTES

IS THIS TEA GOOD ICED?	PURCHASED FROM	
☐ yes ☐ no		
WOULD YOU BUY AGAIN?	IDEAL FOR	RATING
☐ yes ☐ no		☆ ☆ ☆ ☆ ☆

TEA TASTING NOTES

DATE	TEA (NAME/BRAND/SELLER)	
COUNTRY OF ORIGIN:		PRICE

TEA TYPE

☐ black ☐ green ☐ white ☐ herbal ☐ oolong ☐ pu-erh ☐ fruit ☐ other

BREWING METHOD	DRY LEAVES (AMOUNT)	WATER TEMP.	STEEPING TIME(S)

TEA LEAVES	LIQUOR (COLOR)
AROMA	LIQUOR (TASTE)

AROMA CHECK LIST

☐ bitter ☐ robust ☐ nutty ☐ earthy ☐ citrus ☐ flowery ☐ sweet ☐ delicate ☐ malty
☐ spicy ☐ woodsy ☐ smokey ☐ other

PREPARED WITH

☐ sugar ☐ milk ☐ cream ☐ lemon ☐ honey ☐ other

NOTES

IS THIS TEA GOOD ICED?	PURCHASED FROM	
☐ yes ☐ no		
WOULD YOU BUY AGAIN?	IDEAL FOR	RATING
☐ yes ☐ no		☆ ☆ ☆ ☆ ☆

www.ingramcontent.com/pod-product-compliance
Lightning Source LLC
Chambersburg PA
CBHW071421070526
44578CB00003B/649